How to Live with Diabetes

How
to Live
with
Diabetes

Fourth Edition

HENRY DOLGER, M.D.

and BERNARD SEEMAN

SCHOCKEN BOOKS · NEW YORK

First published by SCHOCKEN BOOKS 1978

Published by arrangement with W. W. Norton & Co., Inc.

Copyright © 1977, 1972, 1965, 1958 by Henry Dolger and Bernard Seeman

Manufactured in the United States of America

Contents

Foreword

This is a book for diabetics and for those relatives and friends of diabetics whose lives may be touched by the disease.

Its major emphasis is on the person with diabetes rather than on the ailment or condition. While it deals with the questions of diagnosis and treatment, the book is more concerned with the human factors, the problems of daily living as they relate to growing up, work, marriage, sex, aging, and the means of adjusting to the numerous physical and emotional demands of the disease.

These matters are examined in detail and discussed realistically on the basis of day-by-day experience with thousands of diabetics of all ages.

In the main, attention is directed to those phases of the disease which the patient can help control. Certain complications which cannot be influenced by any direct contribution on the part of the diabetic are omitted.

This is no do-it-yourself manual and makes no effort to show the diabetic how to treat the disease on his own. Instead it is designed to help the reader understand diabetes on a medical as well as on a personal level. It deals with the medical aspects of the disease—its development, course and vagaries—so that the reader will be able to appreciate the principles behind the treatment prescribed by the physician and why sudden changes in treatment may be ordered.

The new oral drugs are discussed in detail; their characteristics, the areas in which they are useful, their modes of action insofar as these are known, and the dosage forms now available. Moreover, note is taken of the controversy that has arisen in the United States regarding their possible hazards.

Also described are the newer concepts of diabetes as well as current research into the possible causes and the nature of the ailment, its detection prior to the appearance of overt symptoms (the "prediabetic" state), and the developing possibilities of diabetes prevention.

Since it is assumed that the diabetic is under medical care, the chapter on diets presents none of the currently used diet prescriptions. Where diets are used in treatment, they should be left to the judgment of the attending physician.

Altogether, the function of this book is to help the diabetic live with his disease. This requires the fullest possible understanding of the ailment, the medical principles underlying its management, the problems it imposes on the patient and his family and how these problems may be met.

Such an understanding should help arm the diabetic to face his disease on the best possible terms.

HENRY DOLGER, M.D.

New York, N.Y.

How to Live with Diabetes

PART ONE

The Disease

CHAPTER 1

What About Diabetes?

"Will I live?"

That is the first question a doctor usually hears when he tells a patient he has *diabetes mellitus*.

Then come other important questions.

"Will I be able to keep working?"

"Will I have to change my way of life?"

The answers are different today from what they would have been, say, in 1920. Given the benefits of modern treatment, the diabetic *can* live a normal life in virtually every respect. He can work, play, even be a parent. He can do almost everything the non-diabetic can do. But first, he must learn to live with his disease.

The diabetic should know everything that can be known about his ailment, its history, nature, how it develops, the problems it creates, how it is treated. He should understand the reasons for treatment. He should be able to distinguish medical fact from popular fancy, prejudice from sound practice. Knowing these things, he will be better able to cope with his disease every day of his life.

Diabetes mellitus is a metabolic disease. As far as we know, it is not caused by bacteria, viruses, or other microbes. It does involve an inability on the part of the body to perform certain vital functions. As a result, the diabetic is unable to use the carbohydrates he eats, the sugars and starches, and turn them into the heat and energy his body needs to operate normally.

The Search for a Cause

Although diabetes is one of the oldest diseases known to man, its actual cause is unknown. Almost 3,500 years ago, a medical scribe of ancient Egypt described the disease in a manuscript now known as the Ebers Papyrus.

Physicians of ancient Greece also knew about this disease, and it was they who named it *diabetes* which means "siphon" in Greek. This refers to one of the most prominent symptoms of the ailment—frequent urination.

It was not until late in the seventeenth century that the adjective *mellitus* was added to the name to distinguish it from another disease named *diabetes insipidus*. *Mellitus* comes from the Latin word for honey and it refers to the fact that diabetics have sugar in their urine.

Early diagnosis involved tasting the urine. If it was sweet, the patient had *diabetes mellitus* and could expect about five to ten years more of life.

In 1783, an English physician, Thomas Cawley, became the first to record a diagnosis of *diabetes mellitus* by showing the actual presence of sugar in the urine. Five years later, while performing an autopsy, Cawley discovered an important clue to the possible cause of diabetes. He noticed that the pancreas, a gland just below and behind the stomach, seemed different in a diabetic than in a healthy person.

Cawley reported this observation but disregarded it himself since he was already convinced that diabetes was a disease of the kidneys. Perhaps if early records had been better kept or if scientific communication were on a more efficient level, Cawley would not have dismissed the importance of the pancreas. He might have known that in 1682 it had already been suggested that the pancreas was necessary for the complete utilization of carbohydrates.

Then, about 1860, Étienne Lancereaux, a Paris physician who had done considerable work with extremely emaciated diabetics, stated his conviction that diabetes *was* the result of a disordered pancreas.

The controversy continued to rage. While there were many theories about what started the disease, nothing very effective could be done to treat it, and the patients generally died. Still, reasoned the doctors, once the cause could be pinned down, the cure would logically follow.

A century after Thomas Cawley made his observation regarding a pancreatic change in a diabetic, two doctors performed an epoch-making experiment and stumbled upon an important fact as a result: In 1889, J. von Mering and O. Minkowski succeeded in removing the pancreas of a dog. In view of the fact that the dog survived the experiment, this was a remarkable feat.

Then the unexpected happened. The dog began to urinate with abnormal frequency, and clouds of flies gathered wherever he urinated. Bernhard Naunyn, von Mering's and Minkowski's medical superior, noticed this phenomenon and suggested that they analyze the dog's urine. They did and found that it contained sugar.

By removing the pancreas of the dog, the two doctors discovered that they had created a condition that duplicated diabetes in man. Step by step the diabetes symptoms developed until the animal passed into diabetic coma and died.

The discovery that removal of the pancreas resulted in diabetes did not produce a cure. So the search went on.

Meanwhile, a brilliant German medical student, Paul Langerhans, had made a remarkable advance. In the pancreas he found clusters of cells completely unlike the ordinary tissue of the gland. The purpose of these cells was still to be revealed, but they were given a somewhat romantic name—the islets of Langerhans. ·

Determined to find which part of the pancreas might be involved in diabetes, medical researchers continued their investigations. They tied up the main duct of the pancreas so that the gland shriveled, leaving only the islets of Langerhans intact. *This produced no diabetes.* But when the shriveled gland was removed *together with* the islets of Langerhans, *diabetes was produced.*

Was there something in the islets of Langerhans which made sugar metabolism possible—without which diabetes resulted?

It was while trying to find an answer to this question in 1921 that F. G. Banting and C. H. Best of Canada made their great discovery. It earned Banting a Nobel Prize and a knighthood, and gave the world the first effective means of treating diabetes.

The discovery was insulin, a hormone normally produced in the islets of Langerhans, which permits the body to metabolize sugars and starches and convert them into heat and energy.

The first human patient was a Toronto physician, Joe Gilchrist, who had severe diabetes. The results were described as "excellent."

Although the isolation of insulin provided a treatment for diabetes, it did not solve the problem of the underlying cause. Some people become diabetic even though their production of insulin is normal. Examination of diabetics killed in automobile accidents show some to have adequate concentrations of insulin in the pancreas.

Several Causes Seem Likely

In every case of diabetes there *does* seem to be some impairment of the insulin mechanism—either in its production or the way it works in the body. This has led scientists to suspect that what we know as *diabetes mellitus* may be several different diseases, each producing an inability to utilize carbohydrate due to insulin malfunction.

There are at least five factors which may interfere with normal insulin activity and thus produce diabetes:

1. There may be an inability on the part of the beta cells of the pancreas to produce enough insulin because the pancreas is diseased or absent. Should the pancreas be damaged or destroyed by a tumor, or removed by surgery, diabetes invariably results.

2. There may be an increase in the rate at which the body uses up insulin. This may be caused by overeating or by overactivity of the thyroid gland. Where this creates an insulin shortage, diabetes results.

3. There may be an increase in the rate at which insulin is destroyed in the body. There may be a drop in insulin production, or its effects might be inhibited by the action of certain body chemicals. These chemicals include such enzymes as insulinase as well as insulin antibodies and certain proteins which attach themselves to insulin and inactivate it. In addition, the body may even produce abnormal insulin which is unable to fulfill its role in carbohydrate metabolism.

4. There may be a drop in the efficiency of insulin due to the introduction of certain chemicals which impede insulin activity. These include cortisone and its derivatives, ACTH, purified growth hormone, isonicotinic hydrazide, large doses of nicotinic acid, and certain diuretic drugs such as the thiazides which are used to

rid the body of excess fluids. Even the birth control pill has come into question as having a possible effect upon sugar tolerance, but this has not been proved. There may also be other drugs, used to treat various diseases, which can affect insulin activity.

5. In the alpha cells of the pancreas, the body produces a hormone which has an effect opposite to that of insulin. This substance is called *glucagon,* and it acts to release glucose from the liver into the blood. Normally, glucagon might thus help the individual survive during periods of starvation. However, the release of abnormally large amounts of glucagon appears to have a role in diabetes.

6. The delta cells of the pancreas release a hormone called somatostatin which is also produced by the hypothalamus, at the base of the brain. This hormone seems to have a regulatory function and serves to maintain a balance between insulin and glucagon by inhibiting their release. Should there be any abnormality of somatostatin production or activity, the insulin-glucagon equilibrium will be upset and diabetes may result.

7. Recent research has shown that insulin and glucose attach themselves to specific locations on the body cells. These are known as receptor sites. If they are defective or inadequate in number, insulin will not perform its task, glucose will not enter the cell but instead remain in the blood, and diabetes can result.

8. Viruses may have a role in causing some diabetes. Scientists have shown that certain viruses can damage or destroy the insulin-producing beta cells in experimental animals. There is also evidence that similar viral damage can be done to humans.

Any or all of these factors, as well as others not yet discovered, may bring about the set of symptoms we call *diabetes mellitus.* But the underlying cause or causes are still unknown. There are a number of theories but no conclusive proof.

Just as the cause of diabetes remains a mystery, so does the manner in which insulin works. Biochemists produce enough insulin to treat all diabetics who need it, but how this protein substance helps the body turn sugar into energy remains a puzzle.

At present there are three major theories, each of them involving complicated biochemical processes. One thing *is* certain about insulin, however. Scientists may not agree on *how* it works, but there is no disagreement about the fact that it *does* work, making it possible for a diabetic to live a fairly normal life.

But fairly normal does not mean perfectly normal. The diabetic faces hazards not common to the non-diabetic. There is a greater susceptibility to certain infections and ailments. There is a speeding-up of certain degenerative processes—especially in the eyes, kidneys, circulatory and nervous systems.

With proper care and careful hygiene some of these hazards may be controlled and held to a minimum. This must begin with prompt diagnosis—detecting the disease as soon at it appears.

The classical symptoms of diabetes, detailed in Chapter Three, are easy to recognize and show themselves in most, but not all, cases.

The majority of cases can be recognized readily enough by the physician, and while a few may present diagnostic problems, there is no reason why any diabetes should remain undetected and untreated.

The Meaning of Metabolism

Before we go any further into the details of diabetes, we should have a clear picture of what metabolism means to us. Unless we understand the metabolic process, the idea of a metabolic disease will be hard to grasp.

All of us must eat and breathe in order to live. Eating provides us with nutrients such as carbohydrates, proteins, fats, minerals, and vitamins. Breathing provides us with oxygen.

The nutrients we eat and the oxygen we breathe are used by the body to make possible all the countless physical and chemical activities necessary to life.

Two fundamental processes are involved in metabolism. One is known as *anabolism*. The other is *catabolism*.

Anabolism means building up. The simple chemicals into which our foods have been reduced by digestion are rearranged and built into substances the body needs— new cells, tissues, blood, bone, muscle, and other material necessary to health and life.

Catabolism means breaking down. Worn-out or damaged cells and tissues of the body, materials that have served their purpose and are no longer needed, are broken down into simple chemicals. Depending upon the needs of the body, these may be eliminated as waste or rearranged and used again in some other form. In the various stages of catabolism, energy is released.

These two processes of metabolism are continuous whether we are at work or at rest, awake or asleep. But the tempo at which they operate keeps changing as the demands upon our bodies change with stress, activity, growth, illness, or aging.

For proper health there should be a balance between the foods we eat and the metabolic needs of the body.

If we eat too little food, the body turns upon itself and breaks down its own tissues—fats and proteins— to provide energy and chemicals for essential life functions. This is what happens when we go on weight-reducing diets. Carried to extremes, it results in starvation.

If we eat too much food, the excess is converted into

fat which the body stores away. This results in overweight and obesity.

Our food needs and metabolic activity are highest in infancy, childhood, and adolescence, since that is when we have the greatest rate of growth. As we get older and stop growing, the food intake must be reduced to match the decreasing need.

With old age our energy needs decline, causing a. progressive slowing of our metabolic tempo. So our food needs diminish further. This is why elderly people may put on excess weight although they eat no more than before.

By viewing metabolism as a continuous process that provides heat, energy, and living substance from the food we eat and the air we breathe, we can see that without metabolism there can be no life, and with faulty metabolism there can be no health.

When a person get *diabetes mellitus*, a very important part of the metabolic process breaks down. What happens as a result is similar to what happens in starvation, and many of the symptoms are the same.

Where the starving person can use carbohydrates but does not have them, the diabetic has them but cannot use them. The outcome is the same, but for one major difference. In the diabetic, the unused sugar piles up in the bloodstream and body tissues, then "spills" over into the urine. The kidneys work continuously to get rid of the excess sugar. This drags water out of the system and causes dehydration and insatiable thirst.

Since the body needs energy to live, and the usual foods do not provide it, the body begins to consume itself. This process, the same in diabetes as in starvation, is not very efficient in energy production. As it continues, dangerous by-products of fat metabolism are formed.

Known as ketone bodies or acetone, these chemicals

are poisonous to the system in large quantities. They accumulate in the bloodstream, pour into the urine and, as the diabetic becomes less able to handle the rising ketone level, acidosis sets in. This is followed by coma and, finally, death.

That would be the course of diabetes if left untreated. And, before the isolation of insulin in 1921, diabetes was almost invariably fatal.

We have come a long way in the last few decades—more than the preceding thirty-five centuries. Diabetes may still be almost as much a mystery as it ever was, but it is no longer as big a problem.

This does not mean that diabetes is on the decline. It does mean that we are at last able to live with it. In view of the fact that more of us can expect to become diabetic as our life span increases, this represents substantial progress.

CHAPTER 2

Who Gets Diabetes?

Practically anybody can get diabetes, regardless of age, sex, race, or social station.

Unlike polio, tuberculosis, and pneumonia, diabetes is not on the wane. Instead, it grows more prevalent as it reaches out to mark an increasing number of people each year.

Recognizing the scope of the problem, the United States Congress mandated the National Commission on Diabetes to prepare a long-range plan to combat diabetes mellitus. The Commission estimated that in 1975 ten million Americans were directly affected by diabetes. One of every five Americans born that year, they declared, will develop diabetes if he or she has an average life span of 70 years.

As for the toll of the disease, the Commission reported that, in 1975, 38,000 persons died directly from diabetes, and its economic cost was estimated to be $5.3 billion annually.

What is more, during the next few decades the rate of increase in the number of diabetics in this country will be more than four times greater than the rate of increase in the total population.

The youngest diabetics ever recorded were a brother and sister. The girl became diabetic at the age of 4 months. Her infant brother was diagnosed as a diabetic at the age of 9 days. Today, almost ten years after the onset of the disease in the boy, both children receive small amounts of insulin daily and are growing normally.

Diabetes has been called a disease of old age. This is not strictly true. While 80 percent of all diabetics are over 40 years of age, there is also a considerable incidence of the disease in childhood, adolescence, and young adulthood, with about 5 percent of all diabetics being of the juvenile-onset type.

In Britain, the Bedford Survey estimated that there are 200,000,000 diabetics in the world and that 14.5 percent of the individuals over age 50 are diabetic.

In the United States, however, a long-term study in Tecumseh, Michigan, suggested that 30 percent of the population over age 60 has either overt or chemical (asymptomatic) diabetes.

As far as age is concerned, we are vulnerable to diabetes throughout our lifetimes. There is a gradual increase in susceptibility, with slight peaks at puberty and during pregnancy, until we reach the age of 40. Then there is a rapid jump.

Females Are More Susceptible

Diabetes overlooks neither sex but it *does* seem to have a special preference for women except among certain ethnic groups such as the East Indians of Natal, South Africa, and some American Indian tribes. Among these peoples, men have a higher incidence of diabetes. During childhood, adolescence, and young adulthood, the disease plays no favorites between the sexes. At the age of 30, the woman becomes more susceptible until, between 45 and 65, she is twice as likely as a man to get the disease. A striking increase in susceptibility occurs as the woman approaches the menopause.

One of the most unusual aspects of the disease is the

apparent link to marriage and motherhood. The highest number of deaths from diabetes is among married women —and this includes widows and divorcées. The death rate among married women is almost twice as great as among single women.

The married man is far less susceptible than the married woman. For him, the wedded state acts as a protection, and his death rate from diabetes is lower than that of bachelors, widowers or divorcés.

Why should women be more susceptible to diabetes than men, and married women more than single women? Motherhood seems to be the reason. The woman with more children is more susceptible than the women with fewer children. The more pregnancies a woman undergoes, the greater is the possibility that she will become diabetic.

In 1949, three Scottish doctors, H. N. Munro, J. C. Eaton, and A. Glen, completed a thorough survey on the subject in a Glasgow Diabetes Clinic.

Obesity and heredity are ordinarily considered major factors in diabetes susceptibility. The increased susceptibility of married women has been attributed to the fact that they are frequently overweight during and after pregnancy.

To check this theory, the Scottish doctors studied a number of women of comparable obesity and found that the tendency toward diabetes varied directly with the number of children each woman had borne. The highest incidence was among the women with the biggest families.

As for the influence of heredity, the doctors found that women with six or more children were likely to get the disease even where there was no history of diabetes in the family.

These studies were conducted carefully to make a clear division between obesity and heredity on one hand, and frequency of motherhood on the other. The results showed that childbearing, by itself, must be considered an important factor in the development of diabetes among women.

Still another element in diabetes susceptibility is the size of the infant a women bears. Not long ago—and in some areas even today—many parents felt that a bigger baby was a healthier baby. Today we know that an infant's size is no measure of its health, and the bigger the infant, the greater the likelihood that the mother will become diabetic. The woman who bears a child weighing ten pounds or more has a greater than 75 percent chance of becoming diabetic.

Thus, the reason for the sharp rise in diabetes among women over 40 seems mainly due to the stress of repeated pregnancy plus the dynamic upheaval of the menopause.

Race and Nationality Are Not Factors

A number of theories have linked diabetes to race, nationality, and geography. Negroes, for example, were supposed to have less diabetes than whites; Chinese and Japanese, less than Europeans.

The reason Southern Negroes appeared to have less diabetes was because they were less likely to have proper medical treatment, and less diabetes was therefore diagnosed.

In urban areas, where medical care and diagnosis are more easily available, existing diabetes is more frequently recognized and reported than in rural areas. These factors, not race or nationality account for, say, the apparently higher rate of diabetes among Jewish people, concentrated, as most are, in cities. And in the cities of the North, diabetes is just as frequent among Negroes as among whites.

In areas where there is marked undernutrition and semi-starvation, there is less diabetes. In India, for instance, diabetes is not uncommon; but because of the low-calorie, low-protein, low-fat diet, the disease is usually mild. In the more prosperous, better-fed classes, however, diabetes seems to be more frequent and more severe.

The relationship between diabetes and what, how well, and how much we eat is remarkable. During the war, as food restrictions and rationing increased, the severity of existing diabetes decreased; the incidence of new cases declined.

Changing cultural and economic factors have their effect upon diet and stress patterns and thus also influence the incidence of diabetes. This can be seen among the Yemenite Jews now in Israel. These people had a relatively low rate of diabetes when they came as new settlers. After two decades, having acquired a Western life style and diet, their incidence of adult diabetes has risen to about 75 percent of the rate seen in Jews of European origin, and the rate of juvenile diabetes has doubled.

By far the highest incidence of diabetes is among the Pima and Papago Indians of the southwest United States. Among these tribes, according to reports from the Phoenix Indian Medical Center in Phoenix, Arizona, the diabetes rate is 72 percent, 10 to 15 times higher than in the white population. An exceptionally high frequency of diabetes is also being reported from some 41 Indian tribes which also show a greater incidence than whites of cardiovascular complications, and of pregnancy problems such as intrauterine and neonatal loss of babies.

The Phoenix data seem to suggest that this high rate

of diabetes among American Indians is due to underlying genetic factors set into motion by such environmental factors as diet, obesity, and stress.

Among American blacks, the incidence of diabetes is also higher than among whites, matching their high rate of hypertension. This incidence is apparently higher than among African blacks. Thus, in addition to hereditary factors, many environmental factors—a number still unrecognized—must certainly be involved.

Actually, diabetes is virtually universal. After the Pima and Papago Indians, the East Indians of Natal have the highest rate, with 42 percent of all adults being diabetic. The Chinese, Japanese, Malay, and, with one exception, all peoples on earth are vulnerable to diabetes. The sole exception are the Eskimos, who seem to lack the chromosomes for both diabetes and asthma, making both of these diseases extremely rare among them. This would appear to underline the importance of the genetic factor in the evolution of diabetes.

Obesity and Diabetes

Obese people are more susceptible to diabetes than those of normal weight. Where food intake is greater than the metabolic need, the possibility of diabetes increases. This is true regardless of race, nationality, geography, or whether one lives in the city or the country.

Recent research has established that in obese persons the entry of glucose into the cells is impeded because of reduced receptor function at the cells. For this reason, obese individuals have to make more insulin than the nonobese in order to achieve the same effect. Thus, because the insulin is used less efficiently, a greater stress is placed upon the insulin-producing mechanism, accounting for the fact that obese adults often have higher than normal insulin levels in their blood prior to the development of diabetes.

Nevertheless, as Dr. J. Roth of the National Institutes of Health has shown, when obese individuals lose weight, their receptor function improves and their insulin efficiency rises. While these changes vary from individual to individual, they account for the improvement one sees in adult diabetics treated with diet and weight loss alone, one of the oldest approaches to therapy.

Harmful as obesity is to the non-diabetic, for the diabetic it is hazardous to the point of possible catastrophe. Because diabetes results from an inability to metabolize sugars, there is a popular belief that healthy people who eat excessive sweets tend to get diabetes. Yet some of the countries which have the highest sugar consumption seem to have lower diabetes records. On the other hand, the Natal Indians, working on sugar plantations and taking about 30 percent of their nourishment in sugar cane, have an exceptionally high diabetes rate.

Some researchers show that there *is* a relationship between the amount of fat in the diet and the tendency toward diabetes. But the really big dietary factor is not so much *what* you eat as *how much* you eat.

Actually, the type of food is not as important as the amount eaten. Vegetarians get diabetes; people with as varied diets as Japanese, Arabs, and New Englanders get diabetes. Any diet, if it results in weight gain and obesity, will be diabetes-inducing. Any diet which reduces weight —Weight Watchers, the Drinking Man's Diet, or any other—will tend to either diminish the likelihood of diabetes or make it less severe.

While obesity is today accepted as the most common precipitating factor in diabetes, this does not imply that every overweight person—or even the majority of them —will become diabetic. But at least three of every four adults who became diabetic were overweight before they developed the disease.

Heredity and Diabetes

If obesity is the most common *precipitating* factor in diabetes, heredity is the most important *predisposing* factor. Where genetic susceptibility is present, any of the stresses—obesity, disease, pregnancy, steroids, high-carbohydrate diet, and so on—may induce diabetes. If there is no genetic susceptibility, diabetes is unlikely.

The influence of heredity is often a very elusive element. A diabetic may prove to a doctor that neither his parents, grandparents, nor great-grandparents had diabetes. This still would not eliminate the possibility of a hereditary predisposition. Many people who are latent diabetics may die from other causes *before* the disease develops. Children of these people may be predisposed to diabetes although their parents would seem to have been non-diabetic.

There is a wide difference of opinion regarding the rate of genetic transmission of diabetes. Dr. D. L. Remoin of St. Louis believes that the offspring of two diabetic parents have a 1 percent chance of developing diabetes before age 20, whereas Priscilla White of Boston claims the likelihood to be between 25 and 30 percent. Clearly, while there is no question about the fact of heredity susceptibility to diabetes, the precise nature of its statistical impact is still to be determined.

A final word about heredity. If we take the available facts into account, it would appear that in any tightly knit community or group where there is considerable inbreeding, the diabetes statistics are likely to go up.

There are several other factors in diabetes which should not be overlooked. Some ailments, particularly certain disturbances of the endocrine glands, may be responsible for an onset of diabetes.

Acromegaly, a disorder due to growth hormone over-production; an overactive thyroid; tumors of the adrenal glands; pheochromocytoma; and the use of cortisone all seem to influence our susceptibility to diabetes.

Children who become diabetic are usually taller and heavier than average. This suggests a possible connection between juvenile diabetes and an excessive release of growth hormone from the anterior pituitary gland.

Obesity is also believed to be a factor in juvenile diabetes. This is supported by evidence from Japan, where young boys of about 15 are selected to become the ultra-heavy Sumo wrestlers. These youngsters are fattened up, literally stuffed with food, as part of the training process, and almost all of them are diabetic by the time they reach age 35. In their case, certainly, induced obesity seems to induce diabetes.

Victims of certain viral infections, as well as people subjected to stress and severe emotional upheavals, may find themselves more likely to develop diabetes. This likelihood is further increased if they have any inherent tendencies toward the disease. And in existing diabetes, these factors will unquestionably aggravate the disease.

Now let us return to the question asked at the head of this chapter:

Who Gets Diabetes?

Practically anybody can get diabetes, but an adult is more likely to get it than a child.

A person of a diabetic family is more likely to get it than a person of a non-diabetic family.

An overweight adult is more likely to get it than a person of normal weight.

A person between the ages of 45 and 70 is more likely to get it than a person in any other age group.

Non-whites are 20 percent more likely to get it than whites.

A woman is more likely to get it than a man.

A married woman is more likely to get it than an unmarried woman.

A mother is more likely to get it than a non-mother.

A mother of more children is more likely to get it than a mother of fewer children.

A mother of larger infants is more likely to get it than a mother of smaller infants.

On the basis of all this, the most likely candidates for diabetes are women, particularly non-white women, between the ages of 45 and 70, who come from diabetic families and are overweight.

Of these, the greatest susceptibility of all lies with the mothers of many "king-sized" infants.

CHAPTER 3

The Development
of Diabetes

The classical symptoms of diabetes are so obvious that it should be impossible to miss them. Yet too many people either are unaware of the signs or refuse to recognize them for what they are. The result—for every four known cases of diabetes, about three are undetected and untreated.

Here are the four most important symptoms of diabetes:

Frequent, copious urination.
Abnormal thirst.
Rapid weight loss.
Weakness and lassitude.

Other symptoms include:

Drowsiness and fatigue.
Hunger.
Itching of the genitals and skin.
Visual disturbances, blurring, etc.
Skin disorders such as boils, carbuncles, and infections.
Pain, neuritis of the extremities, numbness.

When these symptoms begin to appear, a trip to the doctor is clearly called for. A simple urine test will usually indicate the presence of diabetes. The doctor can then confirm the diagnosis with either a blood sugar or a glucose tolerance test.

Often, the classical symptoms do not show themselves. In those cases, some complication arising out of diabetes may provide the first clue. A kidney or circulatory disturbance, a stillbirth or other abnormalities of pregnancy all may be signs of diabetes.

Diabetes varies with the people who have it. The severity and course of the illness may change from person to person; may even change within the same person as the result of some new experience.

Many factors influence the course of diabetes—illness, infection, emotional and physical stress, pregnancy. As a result, mild diabetes may suddenly become severe; stable diabetes may become unpredictable. In one case, loss of weight may seemingly eliminate the symptoms of the disease. In another case, a rapid loss of weight may be a sign that mild diabetes has abruptly turned severe.

Most experts studying the problems of diabetes are accepting the idea that the disease should be defined on the basis of the patient's available insulin. Since diabetes is now recognized as a dynamic, changing process rather than a static situation, it has become easier to understand that some patients become dependent on injected insulin during stress, excitement, or obesity, for example, but become insulin-independent when the instigating situation is corrected. Obviously, these people do make their own insulin, but stress impedes either its production, effectiveness, or utilization. Thus, it would be wrong to classify these patients as permanently insulin-dependent. Instead, by understanding the dynamism of diabetes, it can be seen that the disease process involves interactions between food and activity, obesity and weight loss, heredity and environment, stress and recovery. All of these factors, and probably others, produce changes in metabolic balance that affect the availability of insulin and thus the state of the disease.

Another concept that has recently been introduced is that of the "sick beta cell." This term, used by both George Cahill of Boston and Paul Lacy of St. Louis, expresses the idea that a patient with either absent or poor insulin function may have a malfunctioning beta cell, or, conversely, the beta cell may actually be healthy. This raises two questions: If the beta cell is indeed sick, is it recoverable? If the beta cell is healthy, then what is impeding insulin function at the target cells where it must do its job? Obviously, the more we study diabetes the more we appreciate its complexity.

With so many possible variations, it is not easy to classify the different degrees of diabetes. But some form of classification is necessary and, over a period of years, certain categories have been established. These must never be considered as final because time and the experiences of living may create changes in the diabetic and in the nature of his disease.

There are two common classifications of diabetes. The first is called *juvenile* or *insulin-dependent* diabetes. These patients are prone to develop ketosis, and account for about 30 percent of all diabetes.

The second category is *adult* or *maturity-onset* diabetes which is not insulin-dependent, and patients with this form of diabetes are not prone to ketosis. This group is most likely to be successfully treated with diet, oral agents, or both.

Each of these seems to have certain clear characteristics of its own. *Juvenile* diabetes is the form the disease takes in all diabetic youngsters and adolescents. *But it is not confined to juveniles.* Some adults get it; and a few adults suffering from the milder *maturity-onset* form may suddenly have their disease take a turn to the more severe juvenile or *insulin-dependent* form.

A further refinement in classification has been made by S. S. Fajans of Ann Arbor, Michigan. He reported a type of chemical diabetes in young people that is asymptomatic and does not change for as long as 20 years. Although these patients do not have the apparent symptoms of diabetes, glucose tolerance tests show a mild form of the disease. These young people are producing insulin, and their form of disease seems to have the characteristics of adult diabetes. Fajans has named these patients MODYs (maturity-onset diabetes in young). The youngsters with classical juvenile diabetes, who are insulin-dependent, he calls JODYs (juvenile-onset diabetes in young).

Characteristics of Childhood Diabetes

A fundamental difference between *juvenile* diabetes and *adult* diabetes is in the insulin situation. In *juvenile* diabetes there is an absolute deficiency of insulin. This means that the pancreas does not produce even the minimum of insulin needed for bare survival. Therefore, the insulin balance can only be brought to normal by making up the deficit through insulin injections.

With a few possible exceptions, all *juvenile* or *insulin-deficient* diabetics need insulin injections in order to live. On the other hand, many *adult* diabetics can manage their disease on diet alone or with the addition of oral agents.

There are also other differences. In *juvenile* diabetes, boys and girls are equally susceptible. Obesity is *not* a factor, as in *adult* diabetes. Instead, the juvenile patient is usually underweight when the disease strikes; he is also frequently taller than average.

In children, the onset of *juvenile* diabetes often seems very sudden. Actually, it may not be as sudden as it appears. The disease may have been developing at a slower, undetected rate, when, as is so frequent with children, mumps, measles, chickenpox, or one of the other ailments of childhood steps in. Then, as a result of this other ailment, the diabetes flares up dramatically, seeming to appear out of nowhere.

In children and adolescents especially, *juvenile* diabetes is very unstable. The patient's need for different insulin dosages shifts unpredictably as his blood-sugar levels undergo wide fluctuations. This is due to the fact that the demands of growth impose a need for constantly increasing calorie intake and for more carbohydrates.

Children are also more likely than adults to subject their bodies to greater extremes of physical activity—with more violent bursts of exertion on the one hand and longer periods of sleep on the other.

The diabetic child needs insulin injections from the start of the disease, and the dosage usually increases progressively as the child grows older. When adulthood is reached, the dose becomes relatively stable.

There is one more important characteristic of *juvenile* diabetes—a distinct sensitivity to insulin. The *juvenile* or *insulin-deficient* diabetic responds very sharply to its absence or presence. Too little insulin may bring about an abrupt rise in blood-sugar. Slightly too much insulin may cause too rapid a drop in blood-sugar and bring on an insulin reaction.

Characteristics of Adult Diabetes

The characteristics of *adult* or *maturity-onset* diabetes are quite different from the *juvenile* form. The overwhelming majority of diabetics—some 70 percent—are adults who do not acquire the disease until they have passed the age of 35. Many of them are overweight when the disease becomes apparent.

This form of diabetes usually results from a relative rather than an absolute insufficiency of insulin as in *juvenile* diabetes. The *maturity-onset* diabetic need not have a flagrant lack of insulin. He may even have an ordinarily normal insulin supply. But, because something impedes the action of his insulin supply, he gets less insulin activity than he needs for proper carbohydrate metabolism.

Adult diabetes may be mild, moderate, or severe, depending upon the amount of insulin needed to keep it under control. About half of the cases are classified as mild and do not require insulin injections. These can usually be treated with relatively mild dietary restrictions.

There are a number of overweight diabetics whose insulin production is normal but who overeat to the point where they take in more carbohydrate than their insulin supply can cope with. In many such cases, a return to normal weight is enough to correct the relative insufficiency of insulin and free the patient from the symptoms of diabetes.

About half of the adult diabetics may be of normal weight. They do not overeat to any great extent but they do, for some reason or other, have something wrong with the way their insulin works.

If there is a ten percent impairment of insulin function, this can be equalized by a ten percent reduction in dietary carbohydrate. But if the drop in insulin efficiency is greater than ten percent, additional food reduction would cause underweight, loss of strength and a decline in working ability. Therefore insulin injections or drugs which can be taken by mouth are needed.

All this may seem very cut-and-dried. But even *adult* diabetes, usually more predictable than *juvenile* diabetes, has its surprises.

Take an obese individual who constantly overeats. In order to handle his excess carbohydrates, his pancreas becomes overactive and produces more than the normal amount of insulin. If there is no inherent susceptibility and no great stress, he may go on all his life and never develop diabetes.

On the other hand, if he has a diabetic heredity or if he encounters some great physical or emotional stress, a relative insulin shortage may result. Either the pancreas, though apparently healthy, cannot produce that extra amount of needed insulin, or the available insulin is blocked, perhaps because of receptor abnormalities at the target tissues, or for some other reason. A diet that reduces weight and cuts the excess carbohydrate may restore the balance and eliminate the diabetes symptoms.

Suppose this same person who develops a relative insulin shortage does not treat it, or while treating it, suffers a prolonged illness or other stress. This may cause the insulin-producing cells of his pancreas to overwork, give out, and atrophy, producing an *absolute* instead of a *relative* insulin shortage. In such cases we see obese adult diabetics developing the more severe *juvenile* or *insulin-deficient* diabetes.

Apart from their different characteristics, the two types of diabetes also develop differently.

How Juvenile Diabetes Develops

Juvenile diabetes, when it develops in childhood, should be relatively easy to recognize. Most often it begins with the classical symptoms. Where it is not promptly recognized, the error usually lies with the parents who are either unaware of medical developments or do not have an emotional acceptance of the child.

Bed-wetting is usually the first clue to diabetes in a child. Unfortunately, many parents simply regard this as a behavior disorder which they frequently punish.

The next clue is an insatiable thirst which cannot be quenched even with large quantities of soda pop, water and other fluids.

Then comes extreme hunger, weakness, and weight loss. Growing children should be hungry. But when their normal hunger is intensified, and *they lose instead of gain weight*, the hunger may be caused by diabetes rather than the demands of growth.

By this time, with bed-wetting, thirst, hunger, weakness, and weight loss, the parents should certainly be aware that something is wrong with the child and that an immediate consultation with the doctor is necessary. Altogether too many children are not recognized as diabetic until the disease has become so severe that the young victims are in diabetic coma and need to be hospitalized.

Juvenile diabetics usually have a difficult and complicated problem. The younger the child, the greater and more exacting is the care needed to control the ailment.

Episodes of ketosis and coma are more frequent and more sudden in children because of their lower carbohydrate reserves. And, because of the inexorable demands of growth, children cannot accept food reduction as a treatment. For them, insulin is imperative.

Diabetic youngsters sometimes show a temporary remission of symptoms after the start of therapy. This may last for several months. But the need for insulin invariably returns and, with the rare exceptions where a change to an oral drug is possible, remains permanent.

As the diabetic child grows older and reaches adolescence, emotional disturbances related to the disease are often likely to arise. Various things are involved here—the tyranny of daily insulin injections, the need to eat at rigidly fixed times, the restrictions against candy and other sweets which their non-diabetic friends are free to enjoy, anxiety regarding too much physical activity (which may bring on insulin shock) or too little (which may bring on diabetic coma).

These and other factors arising out of his "difference" from other children—if they are emphasized—may add to the tensions and stress of the diabetic child. This, in turn, may stir up the basic instability of the disease and increase its severity.

As treatment of the disease improves, and enlightenment and understanding grows, more and more juvenile diabetics become adult men and women, carry on active and productive lives, marry and rear families. Measure this against the days before insulin when the juvenile diabetic was doomed to die within two years after the onset of the disease.

How Adult Diabetes Develops

The development of *adult* or *maturity-onset* diabetes is usually less severe and less sudden than *juvenile* diabetes. Also it is usually more difficult to detect.

The disease is often so mild at the outset that the patient may learn of it for the first time during a routine examination required by an insurance company for a policy. As a matter of fact, over 30 percent of *adult* diabetes is discovered in this casual way.

A man feels thirsty and starts drinking large quantities of liquids. He might attribute his thirst to the heat, the fact that he is working hard, or the fact that he is urinating a lot. On the other hand, his frequent urination may be attributed to the fact that he is doing a lot of drinking. So the symptoms of thirst and excessive urination may not be recognized for what they are.

The classical picture of weakness, hunger, and loss of weight are obvious symptoms in about one-third of adult diabetics. Diabetes can and has developed in obese people while they were reducing. The loss of poundage is often gratefully accepted as being due to the reducing effort rather than to the diabetes.

All these and other factors frequently delay the recognition of diabetes in adults. The first clue to the presence of the disease may come as the result of a complication rather than from the diabetes itself.

During World War II, a young American lieutenant advancing through Germany attributed his thirst to the summer heat, and his frequent urination to the enormous quantities of beer he quaffed. But one day he became aware that his sexual urges were almost gone. This promptly brought him to the doctor and it was there that the diabetes was discovered.

Quite a number of patients may first go to a dentist because their teeth loosen or their gums become painful or abscessed. Others may go to a urologist because they think their excessive urination is due to a bladder or kidney infection. Some adults, worried about blurring vision, may go to an oculist. Women, perturbed about a persistent genital itch, may go to a gynecologist.

In all of these cases it may then be discovered that the obvious disorders are the result of diabetes.

Women may first become aware of diabetes during a pregnancy or after a stillbirth. Circulatory, kidney, skin, and other ailments may drive an adult to seek medical advice and so first become aware of the fact that he has diabetes.

There is still a further peculiarity of diabetes which can make it even more complicated and unpredictable than it normally is.

Let us imagine an adult with an inherent susceptibility to diabetes. Under ordinary circumstances, he may not develop his diabetes until he reaches the age of 50. But he has an automobile accident, he contracts a severe infection, his wife divorces him, he loses his job.

Under the impact of a series of stresses, his diabetes arrives at the age of 30. Then, as treatment is begun and takes hold, there may be an abrupt remission. The diabetes will mysteriously vanish, not to appear again until the age of 50 or thereabouts, when it originally may have been due.

Once the adult knows he has diabetes and treatment is begun, the chances are that he can live a relatively normal life. The aim of modern medicine is to make the disease and its treatment as inconspicuous as possible so that its intrusion on everyday living can be kept to a minimum. But the diabetic still must take some extra care of himself.

Young or old, he should try to live a regular life. He should try to keep his weight as nearly normal as possible. If he is being treated by diet alone, he should observe its limitations. If he is insulin-treated, his dosage, food intake, and energy output are all balanced. If any one of these is disturbed, he should rectify the others in order to maintain the balance. If he is treated with oral drugs, he may have greater flexibility but should still avoid any excesses.

The diabetic who is able to keep all these factors under control will still remain diabetic for the rest of his life; but, with limitations, he will be able to function almost as well as the non-diabetic.

Some of the world's notable figures have been diabetic.

Among them, writer-historian H. G. Wells, statesman Georges Clemenceau, artist Paul Cézanne, composer Giacomo Puccini, and political leader Fiorello H. LaGuardia all lived full and productive lives. In certain situations, the course of diabetes and its complications in particular individuals may be closely watched by world governments. Mao Tse-tung, for example, was diabetic, as were Francisco Franco and Abdal Gamal Nasser.

Nor need diabetics be a bar to successful careers in entertainment or athletics. Actress Mary Tyler Moore is diabetic, as are tennis stars Billy Talbert and Ham Richardson, ice hockey star Bobby Clark, and baseball's Ron Santo.

CHAPTER 4

The Search for a Cure

The search for a cure for diabetes has been one of the longest quests in the history of the human race.

It began some 3,500 years ago, perhaps a century before Moses led the Israelites out of Egypt, and to this day the cure is still beyond our reach.

We *have* made progress, but basically all that we have achieved, and that relatively recently, is a means of treating the major symptom of diabetes—the inability to metabolize sugar.

The diabetic cannot be cured of his disease as he might be cured of measles, diphtheria, pneumonia, or jaundice. But he can be treated so that the effects are reduced and the disease itself, while not erased, is kept under control.

This does not imply that a cure cannot or will not be found. But the great problem facing medical researchers has been the fact that they still do not know the cause or causes of the disease. They only know its intermediate effect—that something goes wrong with the insulin mechanism, thus interfering with carbohydrate metabolism.

Curing diabetes or any other disease generally involves knowing and eliminating the cause. There are cases where cures have been stumbled upon before the cause of a disease was known. This may result from a happy accident or after many generations of trial and error.

The English were able to cure and prevent scurvy by including citrus fruits in the diet long before it was discovered that Vitamin C existed or that scurvy was due to a deficiency of this vitamin.

Lucky events like these are rare and, as far as diabetes is concerned, the disease appears much too complicated to be tracked down to a single cause. Many factors are involved—the pancreas, the liver, and the ductless glands such as the thyroid, adrenal, and pituitary. But in all cases the result is approximately the same. Whatever the cause, insulin action is impaired and that, at least, can be treated.

Treatments and even "cures" have almost always existed. But none of these "cures" worked and, until recently, neither did the treatments.

The Ebers Papyrus, which dates from about 1,500 B.C., is one of the oldest of all medical documents. It came into the hands of Georg Ebers in Luxor, Egypt, in 1872 and was completely translated by 1890.

From this manuscript it appears that the physicians of ancient Egypt had at least four "cures" for diabetes. The prescriptions were listed under the following heading:

"A medicine to drive away the passing of too much urine."

Typical of these earliest "cures" was this first one listed in the manuscript:

Prescription:

Cakes	
Fresh grits	⅛
Wheat grains	⅛
Green lead earth	⅛
Water	½

Let stand moist; strain it; take it for four days.

How the Egyptian patients fared under these "cures" is not known. Certainly they were not cured.

Early Description of the Disease

In the second century of the Christian era, a truly remarkable physician known as Aretaeus the Cappadocian —Cappadocia was the name of a mountainous region near the Euphrates River in what is now Turkey—gave an astonishingly accurate account of the disease.

"Diabetes," he wrote, "is a wonderful affection, not very frequent among men, being a melting down of the flesh and limbs into urine . . ."

He went on to describe most of the symptoms and then made a speculation as to the cause.

"The cause of it may be that some one of the acute diseases may have terminated in this . . ."

Today's scientists have pretty much gone back to a similar view—that diabetes does not have a single, direct origin but that it results, instead, from other disturbances in the body.

Another "cure" for diabetes was advanced in the sixteenth century by a physician with the improbable name of Theophrastus Bombastus von Hohenheim. Known as [Philippus Aureolus] Paracelsus, he is recognized today as one of the medical giants of history, with views far in advance of his time.

According to Paracelsus, diabetes was due to the accumulation of a salt in the system. To cure it, he suggested fasting for two days, drinking "Julep" to relieve the thirst and getting rid of the salt.

The years passed. Men and women continued to become diabetic and, whether they remained untreated or whether they took the then-accepted "cure," there was little difference in the outcome. They died, usually within five years after the onset of the disease.

It remained for an English physician of the seventeenth century, Thomas Willis, to bring a measure of scientific

sanity to the search for a diabetes cure. Willis, a man pos-
sessing great powers of clinical observation, took the
trouble to taste the urine of diabetics and described it as
"wonderfully sweet as it were imbued with Honey or
Sugar."

In a book published in London in 1679, Willis wrote
that "it seems a most hard thing in this Disease to draw
propositions for curing for that its cause lies so deeply
hid . . ."

So a circle was completed and the disease which could
not be cured by the Egyptians—although they thought
they had several cures—still could not be cured after several thousand years of observation and countless so-called
remedies.

The First Real Dietary Treatment

It was not until 1796 that the first rational attempt was
made at the treatment of diabetes through diet. This was
an epoch-making step since it did not pretend to cure the
ailment, but sought to make it possible for the diabetic to
live with his disease.

Oddly enough, the advance was made by a military
physician, John Rollo, surgeon general of the British
Royal Artillery. Although the science of nutrition had
not yet advanced to the point where proteins, carbohydrates, and the other nutrients were properly recognized—let alone classified and understood—the Rollo diet
seemed to avoid carbohydrates in favor of proteins. The
diet was, said Rollo, "to consist of animal foods prin-
cipally."

Despite many shortcomings, the dietary approach
opened by Rollo raised the curtain on what was to be—
until the isolation of insulin—the first effective means of
treating diabetes. Until 1922, when insulin replacement

became a new basis for treatment, *diet formed the only useful approach to diabetes care.*

The great majority of diets emphasized deprivation. Some patients were helped by some diets, others were injured. Good or bad, each diet had its zealous disciples who maintained that theirs was the only true way and that the others were, at best, mistaken—at worst, a deadly heresy.

At one time, diabetics were made to drink their own urine as a means of restoring lost sugar. In 1857, P. A. Piorry of France fed his diabetic patients more than a quarter of a pound of candy daily to compensate for the loss of sugar through the urine.

Over a period of years, the treatment of diabetics took on the overtones usually associated with the primitive religious ritual of "mortification of the flesh" as a sort of penance for original sin. Only in this case the sin consisted of being a diabetic.

There can be no question that diet saved many lives. This is particularly true of the diet evolved by F. M. Allen in 1914. The Allen diet involved total restriction of calories and emphasized vegetables cooked in three water changes, bran, and olive oil.

The hardships imposed by such a diet were pathetically illustrated by an emaciated 12-year-old boy, who surreptitiously ate his toothpaste and the birdseed of his pet canary.

The dawn of the insulin era, which provided the first original advance in the treatment of diabetes since the Pharaohs, made it possible to free many diabetics from the dietary rigors imposed by earlier treatments. It permitted the use of a higher carbohydrate intake and released millions of diabetics from the often ritualized masochism of self-denial. It also made possible a longer and more normal life expectancy for the diabetic. *But it is not a cure.*

Insulin injections only treat a symptom of diabetes. This is the absence or inactivity of the normal insulin we need to help us metabolize sugars. The injected insulin replaces the absent insulin or reinforces the inactive insulin, but it does not touch the cause of diabetes. Therefore insulin injections are not the perfect answer except in the rare cases where the patient's pancreas is destroyed or has been removed by surgery.

Doctors Differ over Treatment

Although the search for a cure has been held back by the delay in finding the fundamental causes of the disease, there is still another impediment—the fanaticism which has developed around the various approaches to treatment.

Insulin did, after all, free the diabetic from the rigors of a diet that often caused unnatural hardship. Yet, not only were there some who refused to ease the rigidity of the diet, but there is still sharp division over the choice of diet and the type of insulin that should be used. There is even disagreement as to the goals that treatment should seek to accomplish.

One group of doctors holds that the first object of treatment is to keep the urine free of sugar. This is a traditional approach and has a large, influential following.

Another group of diabetes specialists takes a somewhat different view. They feel it is rarely practical to keep the urine constantly free of sugar because this may require a diet that would make it impossible for the diabetic to share in the normal enjoyment of living. Furthermore, they say, overemphasis of this objective of treatment often saddles the patient with worry, depression, inconvenience, and a sense of guilt.

The doctors who support the second viewpoint feel that the important thing in the insulin-treated patient is to keep the sugar level of the blood within bounds, and that moderate amounts of urinary sugar should not cause undue worry. They hold that modern therapy has reduced the need for a rigid diet since, with insulin, the diabetic *can* metabolize carbohydrates. Furthermore, in most cases the insulin dosage can be adjusted to allow the patient to devote more time to enjoying his meals and less time to worrying about them.

Of course, even these doctors agree that some dietary restriction is necessary, especially in obese patients and where there are complications.

The average diabetic, as he views the extremes of this controversy, might well ask himself:

Did the discovery and isolation of insulin free me from slavery to a diet? Or did it merely add the new inconvenience of insulin injections to the existing hardships of the diet?

The truth is that old habits die very hard, particularly if these habits have become fixed and enshrined.

As with any new treatment, insulin came in for sharp scientific scrutiny and considerable resistance on the part of doctors who wanted to be sure that the insulin worked and that the possible harm it might do did not outweigh the potential benefits. This is all part of a normal and natural process. Too much is at stake—human life—to permit acceptance of anything new without substantial proof of its safety and efficacy.

But insulin ran into a further obstacle, the resistance of the "diet-only" cult of treatment. Then, as insulin established itself as the basis of diabetes treatment, the cultists began to accept it and even developed a new cult around it.

Thus, the inflexible ritual of the daily insulin injection, the veneration of sugar-free urine, the dietary taboos and the sense of sinful guilt on the taking of "forbidden sweets" all became part of the new religious discipline of diabetes treatment. And the physician remained vested with the power to reward the patient with an extra slice of bread or to impose the "penance" of additional dietary restrictions.

Pediatricians Force Easing of Rigid Diet

The first break in the "rigid diet" front came in the 1930s as a result, oddly enough, of the pressure of pediatricians. With insulin already in use more than ten years at the time, pediatricians found that diabetic youngsters still did not grow well as a result of undernourishment. Although they were receiving insulin to help them metabolize sugars, they were not being allowed diets to satisfy the caloric needs of growing children.

The pediatricians began to exert pressure to improve the children's diets, urging a more normal caloric intake. The use of insulin, they maintained, had made dietary improvement possible and there was no longer any reason to cling to unnecessary and even dangerous restrictions.

Under this pressure the diets were modified. Gradually the feeling grew and spread that the diabetic—even the adult diabetic—could be allowed to enjoy more normal nutrition as a consequence of insulin.

Today, while the dietary situation has improved considerably, there is still some resistance to change and the tug of war goes on.

The search for a cure did not end with insulin's isolation—although the hormone is so effective a treatment that, for a time, new research lost a good deal of its urgency. But insulin is not a cure, nor is it the perfect treatment. Some patients resist insulin and need unusually large amounts. It has to be handled carefully and administered in exact dosages. Furthermore, while it may free the diabetic from the unyielding adherence to a rigid diet, it also chains him to the need for daily insulin injections and exposes him to the hazards of insulin shock.

The fact that insulin has to be injected has been a major problem. Since it is a protein substance, it is destroyed by the digestive juices and therefore cannot be taken by mouth. This creates a number of special problems. The diabetic, obviously, cannot be expected to go to his doctor every day for his injection. Consequently he must give it to himself or have some relative or neighbor give it to him. It is easy to see how the need for insulin injections, apart from being inconvenient, may sometimes become a distinct hardship.

So, from the very moment insulin was discovered, a search was begun for a drug which could be taken by mouth to control diabetes.

In June, 1957, after an intensive period of work which had been set into motion as the result of a series of medical accidents, the first substance which could be taken by mouth to reduce blood sugar was released to physicians in the United States. This drug, already widely used in Europe, has the chemical name of tolbutamide and is distributed in this country and Canada as Orinase. In the rest of the world it is known as Rastinon.

While this and other oral drugs are certainly no cure, they can replace insulin injections in many adult diabetics.

Even more important from a scientific standpoint, the oral drugs such as Orinase, Diabinese, Dymelor, Tolinase, and DBI are providing a new surge of inspiration to diabetes investigation. Using these drugs as research tools, scientists have set into motion a tide of fresh investigation.

What they find most fascinating is the possibility that these drugs may help provide the key to the mystery of how insulin works. And this, in its turn, may open the long-locked door to the causes of diabetes and thus, after 3,500 years, bring within reach the possibility of a cure.

Another major advance toward the understanding of diabetes has been the synthesis of the insulin molecule.

In 1960, working independently, a Toronto group under G. H. Dixon and a Shanghai group under Y. C. Du split the insulin molecule into its component parts and then reconstituted it.

Following this achievement, a Pittsburgh team headed by P. G. Katsoyannis completely synthesized the separate A- and B-chains which, together, constitute the insulin molecule. These two chains were then linked by Dixon to form the complete hormone.

This was the first time so complex a molecule as insulin had been constructed by man. The importance of this accomplishment is almost beyond estimation at this time. It makes possible the creation of insulin with built-in radioactive tracers that may provide definitive clues as to precisely where and how this hormone achieves its metabolic effect. It also opens the way to the possible manipulation of the insulin molecule so that forms might be created that could be taken by mouth rather than by injection.

PART TWO

The Management
of Diabetes

CHAPTER 5

Diet and Diabetes

Fifty years ago, the average diabetic faced a gloomy prospect. In severe cases, he usually died after a relatively short illness. In milder cases, he had the choice of a slightly longer life—perhaps five or more years—or, if he were willing to undergo the rigid deprivation of the existing treatment, possibly ten years of something less than life.

Today, with insulin, the new oral drugs, and better general treatment, a diabetic can enjoy a virtually normal life span. The doctor's goal in treating him is not merely to keep him alive but to make it possible for him to live, work, and function as fully as his capabilities permit.

The change that has taken place can be summed up by the catechism for diabetics developed by the late E. P. Joslin of Boston.

Prior to 1922, the question "What are you to do with an apple?" was to be answered, "give it away." Now, Joslin could accept the reply, "Eat it."

Difficult as the early treatments were for diabetics, the fact remains that they were treatments. They were hard on the patient—sometimes unbearable—but in many cases they permitted him to survive longer than would otherwise have been possible.

We have already noted that the first effective dietary approach came in 1796 when John Rollo undertook the treatment of a certain Captain Meredith. The treatment was rigorous, to put it mildly. In view of what the good captain underwent, he deserves almost as much credit for his fortitude as Dr. Rollo does for his superb medical achievement.

Captain Meredith's ordeal began with a bleeding; then, confined to a room, he was placed on the following diet:

"Breakfast, 1½ pints of milk and ½ pint of lime water mixed together; and bread and butter. For noon, plain blood puddings made of blood and suet only. Dinner, game or old meats which have been long kept; and as far as the stomach may bear, fat and rancid old meats, as pork. To eat in moderation. Supper, the same as breakfast."

In addition to this diet, Captain Meredith had his skin greased daily with lard; and an ulceration, the size of a half-crown, was maintained opposite each kidney.

The captain was 34 at the time and his diabetes, which had developed seven months earlier, was moderate. He improved steadily and, as his urine became sugar-free, the strict diet was gradually relaxed to include such vegetables as cabbage, lettuce, boiled onions, and radishes. In due time, Captain Meredith was able to resume his military career.

Early Diets Made Eating Loathsome

Rollo knew nothing of the metabolic nature of diabetes and the fact that it involves a failure of carbohydrate utilization. His diet, based on trial and error with a good helping of intuition, was truly a remarkable advance. In fact, some of the more scientifically founded diets of the twentieth century were modifications of the Rollo diet which emphasized proteins and fats, curbed carbohydrates. It also curbed the total intake of food by making eating as distasteful as possible.

An insight into the theory behind this can be had from

Dr. Rollo's account of two diabetics who, after consuming the lees of oil and drinking melted fat, "contracted so great a loathing of food, that neither of them ate anything for five days, and so got rid of their distempers."

The practice of curbing food intake by making eating unpleasant gathered great vogue in the years following the introduction of the Rollo diet.

Robert Watt of Scotland was one of a number of physicians who gave their patients antimony powders to curb their appetites. The powders, wrote Dr. Watt, "produced very severe sickness, vomiting, and commotion in the stomach and bowels. Anything which produces sickness has a temporary effect in relieving diabetes. . . ."

As the years passed, the strict animal diet with its emphasis on rancidity gradually changed. Apollinaire Bouchardat, one of the great diabetes clinicians of the last century, modernized the Rollo diet. He insisted on individualizing the treatment for each patient, objected to the rancidity of Rollo's fats and substituted fat and alcohol for carbohydrates.

Alcohol, since it requires no insulin, is readily converted into energy and was frequently used to replace carbohydrates in the diet of diabetics.

It was Bouchardat who began the practice of fast-days for diabetics. While he was the first to show the value of the intelligent use of exercise, he injected a religious quality into treatment by telling a patient who asked for bread, "You shall earn your bread by the sweat of your brow."

And the bread which he did allow had to be charred almost to a cinder before he permitted it to be eaten.

Most of the diets of the pre-insulin era were so harsh and restrictive that they were almost impossible to follow. The patients, being human, broke them with enough regularity to impede the treatment. Against this background came the Italian physician, Arnoldo Cantani, who practiced in the second half of the nineteenth century.

Dr. Cantani permitted his patients only lean meat and various fats. In milder cases, eggs, liver, and shellfish were allowed. The total food intake was strictly limited. Cantani felt that about a pound of cooked meat a day was all the food a diabetic needed.

In addition to this, if the urine still contained sugar, the patient had to fast as often as once a week. To make absolutely sure that his patients observed the diet he prescribed, Cantani took the precaution of imprisoning them in locked rooms.

The regular course of the Cantani treatment took three months. If the urine was not sugar-free in that time, the treatment was extended to six and even nine months.

By this time, various dietary schools had come into being, each upholding its particular approach with fierce partisanship. Men like Cantani and his German follower, Bernhard Naunyn, were champions of the rigid carbohydrate-free diet. On the other extreme were the high-carbohydrate schools. These included exponents of milk diets, cereal diets, potato diets, oatmeal diets and a number of others.

By the early part of this century, the partisanship was so intense that some physicians were arguing over the superiority of different brands of oatmeal and the various ways of cooking them.

Science vs. Dogmatism

As these controversies boiled, Naunyn gradually swung away from the extreme Cantani school and developed a diet more closely keyed to the caloric needs and tolerances of the individual patients. But the fast days persisted.

It remained for von Noorden, an eminent diabetes specialist of the era just before insulin, to label these fast days "metabolic Sundays," thus endowing them with an aura of religious self-denial.

Amid all the dogmatism, contradiction and confusion, there were a number of scientists who, instead of upholding this or that diet, were trying to learn more about diabetes.

Notable among these was Rudolph Eduart Külz whose experiments uncovered many errors and superstitions then prevalent among doctors. In 25 years of clinical practice, Külz—who died in 1895 at the age of 50—made a careful study of 1,100 diabetics. Among other things, his experiments showed that a number of drugs widely used to reduce urinary sugar were not only useless but actually harmful. Furthermore, he demonstrated that mineral water had no effect on diabetes. This exploded a delusion that had made diabetics swarm to mineral springs as though they were shrines.

Some of Külz's most important work was in testing the tolerance of diabetics for various forms of carbohydrates. He found that diabetics assimilated starch from green vegetables better than from other sources, that certain forms of sugar—under certain circumstances—were better-assimilated than other forms.

In treating his patients, Külz resorted to neither undernutrition nor fasting. Instead, after testing the amount and kind of carbohydrate each patient could best tolerate, he worked out individualized diets to meet his patient's caloric needs.

While Külz and several other physicians were trying to work out rational approaches to diabetes treatment and were subjecting them to close scientific scrutiny, other doctors went their way enthusiastically promoting their pet panaceas.

The way some of these treatments were worked out

was haphazard in the extreme. The one developed by Guelpa of Paris is a prime example.

The Guelpa treatment was born out of a medical error. A doctor studying the course of typhoid fever made a mistaken observation to the effect that "the more regular and rapid the patient's loss of weight" up to the disappearance of fever, "the quicker and more favorable was his course to recovery."

Although this later proved to be completely wrong, Guelpa seized upon it and applied it first to infections, then to diabetes. His sovereign remedy was to turn the patient into a living skeleton as quickly as possible.

In Guelpa's own words, ". . . the more promptly emaciation sets in, and the more definitely it establishes itself, the more sure and rapid is the patient's progress toward recovery."

To achieve this prompt emaciation, Guelpa subjected his patients to a series of three- to five-day fasts, during which they were copiously purged with cathartics. Between the fasting-purgation periods, the patients were allowed a week to a fortnight of carefully restricted diet which, for the first week, consisted of no more than 2½ pints of milk daily.

This technique of starving and purging patients to the point of emaciation was not confined to the treatment of diabetes. It was also recommended for gout, asthma, rheumatism, anemia, eczema, nervous disorders, insanity, epilepsy, drug addiction, and a number of other afflictions. All this was not a product of the Middle Ages, but part of serious medical practice as late as 1911 and after.

There is even recorded a case, not treated by Guelpa, of an incipient diabetic who fasted for 20 days until his urine became sugar-free.

The Guelpa treatment succeeded in gaining some followers in England and France, and a few favorable results were observed among obese patients suffering from mild diabetes. But in cases of even moderate severity, the treatment was most likely to prove disastrous.

Diabetics Resist Extreme Diets

The normal urge to eat usually conflicted with the treatment. Even patients who willingly accepted restrictive diets—and this included undernutrition treatments less extreme than Dr. Guelpa's—soon found the self-deprivation unendurable. Unless they were locked away or under constant control, they lapsed from the "permitted" to the "forbidden."

A French physician, visiting the United States only a few years before the isolation of insulin, reported that in his country the patients were less willing than those in other countries to accept restrictive diets. Instead, he said, they wanted a diabetes treatment that would permit them to eat freely.

Like the great Athenian orator, Demosthenes, diabetics complained of "the diet prescribed by doctors, which neither restores the strength of the patient nor allows him to succumb."

As more was learned about diabetes, attempts were made to regulate the food intake so that the patient would neither accumulate excess sugar in the system nor toxic amounts of ketone and acetone. These are the metabolic by-products when fat and protein are substituted for carbohydrates as an energy source. Patients on the verge of coma from excess ketone and acetone were taken off fats and proteins and put on a limited carbohydrate diet. When their urinary sugar rose dangerously they were taken off carbohydrates and put on fats and proteins.

This dietary juggling had to be closely controlled in order to adjust for any metabolic fluctuations that might arise. In mild cases, and even in some moderate cases where the patient was obese, diet could be helpful if for no other reason than that it curbed overeating and over-weight. In a number of cases this was able to reduce the patient's food intake to the point where his limited natural insulin supply no longer faced more work than it could handle.

As a result of dietary improvement, the rise in the life expectancy of diabetics was not very great but at least it was measurable.

Herbert H. Marks of the Metropolitan Life Insurance Company, one of the nation's foremost medical statisticians, has shown from the experience of the George F. Baker Clinic in Boston, that during what is known as the era of the Naunyn diet—1897 to 1914—a ten-year-old diabetic could expect 1.3 years of life; a diabetic of 25 could expect 2.1 years; a diabetic of 45 could expect 8.5 years. During the Allen diet era, which lasted from 1914 until 1922, the life expectancy of the 10-year-old had doubled to 2.6 years of life; the 25-year-old's expectancy rose to four years; that of the 45-year-old climbed to 10.5 years.

Allen's Undernutrition Treatment

The Allen diet, worked out by Dr. Frederick M. Allen of the Rockefeller Institute for Medical Research, stands as America's contribution to the treatment of diabetes by systematic undernutrition. In many ways it was a development of the Guelpa semi-starvation treatment.

Under the Allen method, a patient was first fasted for several days, then put on a diet in which carbohydrates, fats, and proteins were all sharply reduced.

In a fairly typical case, treament began with a seven-day fast during which the patient was daily allowed four

bran muffins and some fluids, none of which provided any
calories.

The patient was then allowed to eat for nine days, the
daily calorie total rising from 64 on the first day to 504 on
the ninth. There was a fast on the tenth day and, on the
eleventh day, the patient was allowed 151 calories. With
a fast every seven days, the calorie allowance rose until,
on the thirty-fourth day of treatment, it reached 1,031
calories.

After a patient was discharged sugar-free, he had to
follow a maintenance diet. This involved a fast day, most
commonly every two weeks and usually on a Sunday.
Dr. Allen felt that such Sundays of deprivation would
help the patient in "atoning for any chance indiscretions."

Since the diet emphasized total restriction of calories,
various foods were recommended which offered bulk
without nutrition. One of these foods was bran, a major
part of the bulk in the Allen diet. Dr. Allen suggested
that coarse bran flakes commonly used for the feeding of
cattle were ". . . perfectly satisfactory when washed
under the cold water tap for a half an hour or more . . ."

Indigestible substitutes for flour and other carbohydrates were also suggested. One of these was talcum
powder.

As a possible recipe, Dr. Allen proposed "making a
batter with eggs, spices and impalpable talcum powder,
and frying it crisp. This will appear more satisfying than
the egg fried alone."

Dr. Allen admitted it was possible "for a few cases even
under the most expert care, to end in actual death from
starvation . . ." However he felt that the experience of
Dr. E. P. Joslin showed that death from starvation was
much less frequent than death from coma and was therefore the lesser risk.

This was the high point in the dietary treatment of

diabetes when Banting and Best isolated insulin and began a medical revolution.

For the first time in history, the diabetic patient could be freed from starvation diets. Instead of having to reduce his food intake to meet his limited insulin supply, he could now inject enough insulin to allow him to eat a relatively normal diet without trouble.

That, at least, was the reality made possible by the isolation of insulin. Many doctors were slow to accept this new reality. The dogma of diet was too deeply imbedded to be easily liberalized.

Many mild diabetics can survive without insulin and with relatively minor dietary restrictions. Other patients would require diets that amount to semi-starvation. For them, survival is possible without insulin, but with insulin they could avoid extreme deprivation and live more nearly normal lives. Yet, because of the influence of the diet cult, some of these patients were denied insulin or allowed only enough to make their dietary restrictions barely tolerable. There were even many patients who would rather submit to any privations than take insulin.

For more than ten years after the introduction of insulin, treatment included a subnormal diet until increasing pressure forced gradual reform. Reluctantly, the dietary dogmas underwent modification and, along with these changes, many of the fetishes began to disappear.

Today, although they still have not vanished from the scene, there are fewer diabetics who use special scales to weigh the grams of vegetables or other foods they are permitted to eat; fewer charts on which to enter the records of grams and calories; fewer lists of permitted and forbidden foods.

In about 70 percent of the cases, practical experience has shown that the longer a person has diabetes, the more he tends to deviate from a prescribed diet until a normal food intake is approximated. As a rule, people cannot long be held to a diet that is too different from their normal eating pattern. At the Elliot P. Joslin Camp for Diabetic Boys in Charlton, Mass., 61 percent of the youngsters confessed that they did not follow a diet at home.

A study made in Sweden, where practically all diabetics are registered, bears out the resistance to diets. Only one-third of all those patients who were prescribed diets followed the instructions. The longer a patient used insulin, the more frequently he gradually changed over to a normal diet.

The Modern Diet Returns to Normal

Dietary diehards notwithstanding, it is now generally accepted that the diabetic patient's diet should approximate the nutritional allowances recommended for "normal" people by the National Research Council unless he is overweight or suffers some complication such as hyperthyroidism. In those cases there may be an increase or decrease in nutritional needs.

We also know that earlier estimates of the carbohydrate content of various foods such as string beans, broccoli, and other vegetables were too high because they include indigestible carbohydrates which could not be used by the body. These inaccuracies have been corrected by both the American Dietetic Association and the American Diabetes Association, permitting a somewhat easier diet even for those under rigid carbohydrate restriction.

The physician who treats diabetes today need no longer be a symbol of punishment and deprivation to the patient.

At least 50 percent of adult diabetics can be treated without insulin but with a diet providing a mild to moderate restriction of carbohydrates. Special diets with complicated lists of foods and permissible substitutes are not usually necessary.

Obese patients should have their weight reduced to normal. A 1,200 calorie diet usually is enough to do this. Where a weight-reducing diet weakens a patient, it might be better for him to take insulin or an oral drug and relax the diet.

For diabetics who are not obese and who show little or no sugar in the urine, the simple omission of concentrated sugars, pastry, and soft drinks is often enough. This is especially true of elderly individuals.

The average vigorous adult with mild diabetes and moderate urinary sugar might control his disease by reducing his daily carbohydrate intake and eating adequate fat and protein—meat, fish, eggs, and cheese.

A great number of mild diabetics need not bother with complicated diets at all. They can be treated by omitting from their meals sugars, syrups, pastry, and soft drinks, or by limiting carbohydrates—eating less bread, rice, potatoes, or macaroni. The patient who reduces carbohydrates may increase his protein. The mild diabetic may also use alcohol in the form of cognac, rum, whiskey, or dry wines, since this can be converted to energy by a direct process that does not require insulin.

As far as possible, the diabetic's diet should be kept within the normal pattern of his eating habits. An Italian, for instance, should not be put on a corned-beef-and-cabbage diet.

Currently, a wide variety of foods and soft drinks using saccharine have made it possible for diabetics to enjoy sugar-free foods, drinks, and desserts previously not available to them. Unfortunately, the cyclamates, which afforded better taste appeal than saccharine and permitted many sugar-free jellies and soft drinks to be used without concern for sugar, were summarily withdrawn from sale by the FDA in 1970 in what was considered by many to be an arbitrary action.

Finally, a diabetic who keeps losing weight and does not have the energy he needs to work and live normally should not be treated by dietary restriction alone. He should be permitted to eat the foods that will let him feel and do his best, and be given insulin or an oral drug to help him utilize them.

Juvenile diabetics, especially children, should not have restrictive diets. Only concentrated sugars—soda pop, candy, jams, and jellies—ought to be curbed. Ice cream, cookies, even puddings usually may be eaten. Children need adequate nutrition for proper growth. They must be fed adequately and given enough insulin to help them maintain a positive metabolic balance.

Diabetics of normal weight who take insulin or oral drugs do not usually have to worry about diets. They should not overeat, and they could benefit from a reduction of concentrated sugars. But they are no longer slaves to the diabetic's food scales, food lists, record charts and all the other paraphernalia that once turned the simple act of eating into a ritual involving mathematics, chemistry, bookkeeping, and self-punishment.

This does not mean that the diabetic who takes insulin may eat as he pleases. He must always be on guard to avoid the hazards of insulin shock. Here, the timing of the diet is of paramount importance. Since his daily insulin dosage is specifically geared to the timing and content of his meals, the diabetic *must* eat at the prescribed times. If he wants to avoid trouble he must be sure neither to delay nor skip a meal.

Beyond that, thanks to insulin and the oral drugs, he has been freed from the locked rooms, the starvation diets, the metabolic fasts, and the other mumbo-jumbo of the

Diabetic Dark Ages. He can at last enjoy the simple pleasure of eating without the guilty feeling that he is committing a mortal metabolic sin.

Diabetic diets, when prescribed, have heretofore been complicated affairs involving exchanges by weight of one type of food for another. In order to reduce the dietary complexities, the American Diabetes Association, the American Dietetic Association, and the Federal government are attempting to evolve a simplified approach whereby household measures are used instead of weights, and foods are classified as carbohydrate, protein, or fat according to their main constituent. Thus meat, although it does contain varying amounts of fat, is considered a protein; and bread, which also contains fat and protein, is classified as a carbohydrate. Unfortunately, there are complicated problems attendant upon this attempt at simplification, and more time is needed before they can be resolved.

CHAPTER 6

The Meaning of Insulin

If Otto Folin of Harvard had worked out his test for blood sugar in 1908 instead of 1913, insulin might have been in use 14 years earlier.

History—and medical history is no exception—is as full of bitter ironies as it is of happy accidents. Insulin, or something very much like it, was extracted from the pancreas in 1908 by a German scientist, Georg Zuelzer. This extract was injected into several dogs and the unfortunate animals died. Zuelzer, unable to learn exactly why the dogs died, decided that the substance was too dangerous.

A test would have shown that the insulin extract had caused so rapid a drop in blood sugar that the dogs suffered extreme insulin shock. Even without the blood sugar test, had Zuelzer used diabetic instead of healthy dogs in the tests, his extract would have produced relief of symptoms instead of shock. And Zuelzer would today be one of medicine's immortals, not an obscure scientist whose name is all but forgotten.

Still another rendezvous with immortality ended in a near miss when Israel S. Kleiner of New York and J. R. Murlin of Rochester, N. Y., produced an insulin extract. As with Zuelzer, the blood test that would have shown the importance of the work was not yet available.

Many researchers had already helped pave the way when Frederick G. Banting came upon the scene. Minkowski and von Mering had shown in 1889 that the removal of the pancreas caused a diabetes-like disease in a dog.

In 1900, Opie of Johns Hopkins had reported that in diabetics there was a degeneration in the islets of Langerhans, those mysterious small cells in the pancreas.

Then, in 1916, Sir Edward Sharpey-Schafer speculated that the islets of Langerhans produced a substance without which diabetes would develop. This was the mysterious "X" that scientists were arguing about with great heat; some feeling that it existed and was involved in diabetes; others maintaining that there was no such substance.

Allen, of Allen diet fame, was outstanding among those who opposed the possibility of "organ therapy" and felt that there was nothing in the pancreas that could be used to treat diabetes.

Piece by piece, the evidence continued to mount. There *had* to be something in the pancreas, most likely in the islets of Langerhans, that somehow had a part in the onset of diabetes.

Thus the stage was set for Frederick G. Banting of Canada. In 1920 he was a young orthopedic surgeon who found it so hard to make a living at his profession that he took up part-time teaching at the Western Ontario Medical School.

One evening, while he was preparing a lecture to be given the following day, he picked up a copy of a medical journal and was attracted by an article written by Moses Barron. What he read transformed him from a discouraged young doctor into an inspired researcher. Barron had written that when gallstones blocked the pancreatic ducts, the part of the pancreas that manufactured the digestive juices shriveled up—but the islets of Langerhans were unhurt. Furthermore, wrote Barron, when dogs had their pancreatic ducts tied off the same thing happened. The part of the pancreas that made the digestive juices degenerated, but the islet cells continued to function and the dogs lived.

Banting recalled Minkowski's work. If the whole pancreas were removed the dog died of diabetes. Now Barron seemed to supply the final clue. Where the whole pancreas was destroyed *except* the islets of Langerhans, the dogs *did not* get diabetes and die. Therefore, there had to be something in the islets of Langerhans which, if removed, produced diabetes and death.

The next step was to get at this mysterious substance. Barron had shown the way here too. By tying off the pancreatic ducts of dogs for six to eight weeks, the regular pancreatic tissue would degenerate. Then, removing what was left and making an extract of the still-functioning islets, Banting should have the answer.

The Banting-Best Breakthrough

Banting convinced Professor MacLeod of the University of Toronto Medical School that he had a promising approach to the diabetes problem. With MacLeod's backing and blessing, as well as the facilities of his laboratory, Banting went to work. As an assistant, Banting had a second-year medical student, Charles H. Best, who had, literally, tossed a coin with another student for the job.

It was a grim, heartbreaking task. Failure followed failure. Then, one day in July, 1921, just as they were teetering on the threshold of defeat, came the first glimmer of possible success. Another in a long series of extracts was made and injected into a diabetic dog—and this time the dog miraculously improved. Then it sickened again and died.

Why should the animal die? The answer seemed clear.

One dose of insulin was not enough. The dog had to receive a constant supply of the mysterious substance its own missing pancreas could no longer provide.

In January, 1922, after many more setbacks, Banting and Best achieved what looked like a real experimental success. They were treating a dog—part collie and part just dog—who was diabetic and should have been dead long ago. But the dog, a female, was alive and frisky. The extract worked.

Banting and Best were ready for the really critical test —on a human being. The human guinea pig was Joe Gilchrist, one of Banting's childhood friends. Gilchrist had severe diabetes; and the Allen diet, although it kept him alive, had reduced him to a scant shadow of life.

On February 11, 1922, Joe Gilchrist became the first diabetic human being to receive an injection of insulin. He waited, waited—and then he felt a surge of new life pour through him. The rest is medical history.

Insulin—no longer a hypothetical substance whose existence doctors disputed about—had been isolated, and it worked. A way had at last been found to control the grim course of diabetes—one that would not only keep the diabetic alive but would also allow him to live.

Miraculous though it seemed at the time, the insulin extract used to treat Dr. Gilchrist was far from perfect. For one thing, it was very impure. For another, it was quite unpredictable—getting weaker and weaker in the extract for some unknown reason.

The trouble with the early insulin lay in the extraction process. Banting and Best used a mixture of alcohol and alkali to wash the insulin substance from the prepared pancreas. What they did not know, and neither did anyone else at the time, was that the alkali reacted with the insulin, gradually destroying it.

At this point, a brilliant Canadian chemist, James B.

Collip, appeared on the scene to help Banting and Best improve the purity of their product. Collip not only discovered that the alkali was destroying the insulin, but that it really did a poor job extracting it from the pancreas.

Once he spotted the trouble, Collip substituted an acid for the alkali and tested it. The new alcohol-acid combination fulfilled his expectations. It extracted more insulin from the pancreas and, furthermore, had no destructive effect upon the precious substance.

Diabetics the world over heard of the discovery. Overnight, the demand for insulin went far beyond anything that could be produced from the pancreases of Banting's or any available dogs. Insulin had to be produced in vast quantities to meet the enormous need. There *had* to be some other source.

For a while, Banting and Best were able to obtain an increased amount of insulin from the pancreases of unborn calves. Since the islets of Langerhans formed first, it was not necessary to tie off the pancreatic ducts and then wait for the rest of the pancreas to degenerate. Even with this more accessible source of insulin, the demand quickly outstripped the supply.

At this critical stage, Collip's process provided a solution. His extraction technique made it possible to use the pancreases of cattle and pork *without tying off the ducts.* It also recovered a far greater amount of the available insulin.

First Steps with Insulin

All this time the experimental work went on. Insulin was good, but it had to be made better. Other scientists stepped into the picture. John Abel, a Johns Hopkins

University chemist, was the first to produce pure insulin in crystalline form. This gave scientists a better opportunity to study the newly found hormone.

For diabetics, absolutely pure insulin was no boon. It did not perform at top capacity unless traces of zinc were present. So the zinc which had been purified out of the crystalline insulin was put back in.

The original insulin had no measurement of strength. Since it soon became' necessary to know the concentration being used, an arbitrary measurement was arrived at and called a unit. This was the amount of insulin activity that could lower the blood sugar of a rabbit by a specific amount. This measurement unit is still in use.

When the first commercial insulin, manufactured by Eli Lilly and Co., appeared in the United States, it was very weak, providing only 10 units of activity per cubic centimeter (U10). This regular, unmodified insulin remained active only about four hours and had to be administered before every meal and, in some patients, before going to bed. In 1930, the U10 insulin was replaced by U20, and by 1935 this had been replaced by U40 and U80 insulins, concentrations still available today. But the insulin remained weak, and multiple daily injections were still required.

Meanwhile scientists had been working on methods of prolonging the action of insulin. Various kinds of materials were combined with insulin in order to help slow it down—paraffin, tannic acid, alum. None of them worked.

Different Insulins for Different Needs

Finally, in 1935, a group of scientists under H. C. Hagedorn in Copenhagen announced that they had the answer—two answers, in fact. With this, Denmark began a virtual monopoly on insulin discoveries.

The first discovery prolonged the action of insulin so that one injection could work for 12 to 16 hours. This increase was obtained by adding to the insulin a simple protein substance called protamine, obtained from the sperm of the rainbow trout. The protamine attached itself to the insulin and caused a slower release of insulin activity. This came to be known as protamine insulin.

The second discovery was an extension of the first. Hagedorn found that by adding zinc to the protamine insulin, the action was prolonged even further and would last for more than 24 hours.

Protamine zinc insulin, a milky fluid, was made available in the United States in 1937. With the advent of the Danish-developed insulin, it became possible for most diabetics who needed moderate doses to handle their ailment with only one injection a day.

But protamine zinc insulin did not solve all the problems. There were still a number of diabetics whose insulin needs were so complicated that no one of the available insulins could give them the needed protection with a single injection.

Children, for instance, need very rapid insulin activity. Regular and crystalline zinc insulins gave them the speed they needed but did not last long enough. Protamine zinc insulin did not have a rapid enough onset of action and its duration might be too prolonged, requiring a bedtime snack to prevent an insulin reaction during sleep.

Other diabetics whose disease was erratic found that the protamine zinc insulin did not give enough activity during the day, when they were eating. At night, when the long-acting insulin had no food to work on, there would be too much insulin action and the patient might go into shock.

In the face of these special needs, mixed insulins came into use for juvenile, insulin-deficient diabetics. Instructed by their physicians, the patients would make the mixtures in the hypodermic syringe, combining the required quick-acting and the long-acting insulins to give them the kind of activity they needed.

These mixtures proved so useful, and their use became so widespread that they led to the introduction in 1946 by Hagedorn of Neutral Protamine Hagedorn (NPH) insulin, which also came to be known as Isophane insulin. This insulin has a more rapid onset of action and a somewhat briefer duration of action—18 hours instead of 24. This became a very popular form of insulin, particularly since its onset of action could be made even more rapid with the addition of a small amount of regular insulin into the syringe. A single injection would thus provide rapid morning activity as well as coverage throughout the day, at the same time reducing the hazard of a possible reaction during the sleeping hours. This has been particularly important for children and young adults who are very active.

Two more insulins were still to come. One was Globin insulin, which appeared in 1943 and today is no longer in use. The other and most recent addition to the insulin armory is known as Lente insulin. Developed in 1955 by Hallas-Møller of Denmark, Lente—which means "slowly" in Latin—is a combination of two insulins ⅓ Semilente and ⅔ Ultralente. These, in turn, are made by changing the sodium bicarbonate buffer used in insulins to sodium acetate, providing a slowing effect. Thus, Semilente has a 12-hour duration of action, while Ultralente has a 36-hour duration. The combination of both these, Lente, provides a fairly fast onset of action with a generally uniform 24- to 28-hour duration. For a large part of the insulin-dependent population, NPH and Lente insulins have replaced protamine zinc insulin and the mixtures.

In the eastern United States, the most commonly used insulin today is NPH, which is taken by about 80 percent of the insulin-dependent diabetics, the remaining 20 percent taking Lente. Regular insulin remains in the armamentarium because it is most effective in those situations where very rapid action is needed, as in periods of stress, during infection, and when there is nausea and vomiting. Several injections of this rapidly acting insulin may be necessary during such periods of crisis.

In 1975, when it was apparent that several insulins existed in two concentrations—U40 and U80—and Congress had passed a law to introduce the metric system during the next decade, a decision was reached to make the insulins a uniform U100, while U40 and U80 would be gradually phased out. This made it possible to have a standardized vial for the different insulins, all round. The labels, too, are being made uniform, all in black, and they all have a large, bold letter clearly identifying the type of insulin, R for regular, N for NPH, L for Lente, S for semilente, and U for Ultralente.

Two important advantages are expected to be gained by this standardization of concentration. At present, because of the two different strengths, a considerable amount of insulin is wasted, becoming overage on pharmacy shelves as one or the other strength might be in lesser demand. This waste will be eliminated, because with U100 replacing the other two the pharmacist will be able to carry less insulin. Secondly, the use of only a single-strength insulin, requiring only a single syringe, will tend to eliminate much confusion, particularly the confusion of syringes—using a U40 syringe for U80 insulin, for example. Such an error, which has been a problem for some 40 years, will now be impossible.

The various insulins in this country are made mainly by two manufacturers, Eli Lilly and Co. and E. R. Squibb and Sons. Both these companies derive their insulins from pork and beef pancreas. The insulins from both sources are usually combined, with the percentages varying from season to season depending upon the yield, availability, price and various other factors.

It is also possible to obtain a special insulin upon request from either beef or pork. These can be had as regular, NPH or Lente, making it possible for patients who are allergic to either beef or pork insulin to obtain a form which will not cause an adverse reaction.

Pork insulin, incidentally, is very close biologically to human insulin and is consequently used in patients who, with other insulin, might develop insulin resistance or develop fat atrophy, a condition we will describe later on.

A further improvement in insulin was made by the Danes who developed a technique for the extreme purification of pork insulin so that virtually all impurities have been removed. This is known as single-component insulin. In the United States, improved production methods have resulted in a somewhat similar product, known as single-peak insulin, that is only slightly less pure than the Danish variety.

All insulin now produced by Lilly is the single-peak type, and it is likely that all Squibb insulin soon will also be so. The ultra-purified single-component insulin made by the Danes is available in all types upon special request and at no extra cost. The particular value of these purified insulins lies in the fact that they are virtually non-allergenic and can be used by diabetics who have an allergic response to standard insulins.

Today's diabetic, unlike Joe Gilchrist, has a wide range of insulins at his disposal. None of these is yet the *perfect* insulin. The long-lasting ones do not start soon enough, the quick-starting ones do not last long enough—and all of them have to be injected. Furthermore, while the natural insulin produced by the body is released only to the extent that it is needed at any given moment, in-

jected insulin *cannot* synchronize its activity to the body's
changing blood-sugar levels. Despite these drawbacks,
the total insulin armament is complete enough to provide
an answer to almost every need that may develop in diabetes.

In human terms, the value of insulin and what it has
done cannot adequately be put into words. It made life
possible where there was only the certainty of death.
Even more than bare life, it gave the diabetic that most
precious gift of all—the opportunity to take joy in living.

There is a woman alive today who soon will be cele-
brating 70 years of life. Yet, had it not been for the isolation of insulin, she would most likely have been dead at 15.

Diabetes came upon her suddenly at the age of ten. She
had been a healthy, good-natured child with a fondness
for sweets when the disease struck. In two months, her
weight fell from 64 pounds to 57. The year was 1918 and
there was no insulin, only rigid diet. One year later, after
considerable fasting, she showed some improvement and
was allowed to return to school.

Not for long. Her diabetes became more severe and,
aggravated by an attack of influenza, flared up. Her
weight began to fall sharply and she became bedridden.
By June, 1922, at the age of 14, she was a living skeleton
weighing less than 47 pounds. She had to undergo 5 days
of fasting to avoid passing into diabetic coma.

Three months later she was back in the hospital again
to partake of a possible miracle. If the miracle worked,
she might live. If it did not work . . .

The name of the miracle was insulin—and it worked.

In September she had been taking *no* insulin. Eating
470 calories a day when she was allowed anything at all,
she weighed a shade under 47 pounds and, though nearing
the age of 15, was inexorably withering away.

Three months later, in December, 1922, she was taking

25 units of insulin, eating 1,861 calories a day and weighed 57 pounds. Her once pathetically jutting bones steadily lost their sharpness as the flesh stopped melting away and began to form once again.

In 1969, at the age of 61, having fulfilled the promise of her womanhood as a wife and mother, this once emaciated girl who would otherwise have died at 15 years, succumbed to gastrointestinal cancer in no way related to her diabetes.

Those extra years of worthwhile life give insulin its meaning.

CHAPTER 7

Control with Insulin–
the Tools

Nearly all juvenile-onset diabetics and most young adult-onset diabetics must take insulin. All those suffering from acidosis, disability, continuing weight loss or other complications should take insulin. About half of all maturity-onset diabetics require insulin.

Of the more than five million diabetics in the United States, approximately one and one-half million are being treated with insulin. Another million are controlling the disease with diet, and the remainder are receiving oral drugs.

Since the aim of diabetes treatment is to permit the patient to live as normally as possible, the diabetic who requires insulin is taught by his physician to inject himself. This allows the diabetic greater freedom. Even diabetic children can be taught to handle their own injections.

Infants, the very young, and the disabled cannot inject themselves. In those cases a parent, relative, friend, or neighbor may be required to give the injections. In some unusual circumstances, a nurse or physician may be necessary.

The diabetic who takes insulin has still another responsibility. He must test his urine for sugar, generally at least once a day depending on the nature of his diabetes. He must also be able to test his urine for acetone if the situation requires it.

These tests enable him to keep watch on his condition. If there is any change, the results should promptly be telephoned to his physician, who will then be able to judge what steps to take.

By injecting his own insulin and taking his own tests, the diabetic is free to live his life. Using the telephone as the link with his doctor, he helps make possible treatment by remote control.

Of course, the diabetic must see the doctor for periodic examinations or when there is a change in the status of the disease. Apart from that, as long as he follows the rules of his treatment, he can pretty much go his own way.

In order to be able to handle his own injections, the diabetic must have proper equipment and know how to use it. If a parent, relative, or friend must administer the injections, they, too, must know what to do.

Before we go any further into what the diabetic needs and must know to handle his injections, let us take a closer look at the different insulins and how they act:

The Insulin Armory

Regular Insulin: This is sometimes called crystalline zinc, plain, unmodified, or soluble insulin. It is a clear liquid and comes in round vials with a label marked with a bold, black **R**. Each vial contains 10 cubic centimeters, the standard size for all insulin vials. It is still available in concentrations of U40 and U80, but these are in the process of being replaced by the U100 concentration. Regular insulin is also available in U500 for patients who may need huge daily doses of 200 units or more.

This insulin is quick acting, showing an effect in less

than an hour. It reaches peak activity in three to four hours and activity vanishes in six to eight hours. It is the fastest acting insulin and has the shortest duration. Because of its brief action, this insulin has to be injected before each meal. While it is particularly useful in such emergencies as coma as well as in unstable diabetes where sugar levels shift frequently, it is also being used with increasing frequency in ordinary insulin-deficient diabetes. It is often mixed with longer-lasting insulins to give the latter a fast start.

Protamine Zinc Insulin: A cloudy liquid which *should be shaken until thoroughly mixed.* Instructions on the bottle advise against shaking; these may be disregarded, since experience has shown that proper and complete mixing is essential if the insulin dose is to be uniform. Fresh vials of this insulin should be mixed with special care because protamine zinc insulin has a tendency to clump or adhere to the glass vial after standing for any length of time.

This insulin comes in round 10-cc. vials labeled with a black **P**, and is still being sold in concentrations of U40 and U80, which are being replaced by U100. It is a slow-starting, long-acting insulin with onset of activity in four to eight hours, peak action in 12 to 24 hours and total length of action from 30 to 36 hours or more. Protamine zinc insulin is useful in that small group of patients who need a more pronounced night effect.

Since it has a very long period of action, patients using it may require a light snack before bedtime to avoid possible insulin shock while sleeping. The snack might consist of tea or milk and crackers.

NPH (Isophane) Insulin: NPH, which stands for Neutral Protamine Hagedorn, is a suspension of tiny crystals which, when thoroughly mixed, becomes a cloudy fluid. It currently comes in round vials marked with a large black N, in concentrations of U40 and U80, which are being replaced by U100. In action, it resembles a mixture of three parts regular insulin with two parts protamine zinc. It provides more activity during the day and less at night; begins to act in about four hours, reaches a peak in eight hours and is used up in 24 hours.

This insulin is more flexible, stable, and easier to use than homemade mixtures. It provides insulin action that is closer to the needs of the majority of mild cases and about half the severe cases than do either protamine zinc or globin insulin. Where more rapid action is needed, as with juvenile diabetics, regular insulin may be added to NPH without loss of activity.

Because NPH crystals have an unusual tendency to settle to the bottom of the vial, especially in the cold, this type of insulin may require vigorous shaking to make sure it is evenly mixed. If any crystals are visible, shake thoroughly, even if foaming does result in the vial.

Lente Insulin: This is a combination of two other insulins: ⅓ Semilente and ⅔ Ultralente insulins. Semilente, a suspension of regular insulin, has a rapid action within one to two hours and endures up to 12 hours. Ultralente, a suspension of zinc-insulin crystals, has a very slow starting action and a duration of 36 hours or more. Lente, combining the two insulins, has a fairly rapid onset of action—about one or two hours—and a duration of at least 24 hours. These three insulins come in round vials

labeled with the large black letters of **L** for Lente,
S for Semilente, and **U** for Ultralente, and in concentrations of U40 and U80, which are being replaced by U100.

It may meet the needs of most average diabetics with
a single injection a day as do NPH, or protamine zinc
insulins; and often it also needs a boost of regular insulin
for juvenile and severe diabetics. Lente has been found by
some diabetics to cause a painful or burning sensation at
the site of the injection.

For a number of cases where Lente is not suitable,
Ultralente and Semilente are now available to provide
tailor-made mixtures to fit the patient's special need.

These are the various insulins. Alone or in varying
combinations, they are used to manage those cases of
diabetes which cannot comfortably be controlled by
other means.

The accompanying insulin chart should prove useful
for ready reference:

INSULIN CHART

Type of Insulin	Appear-ance	Identifying Letter	Action be-gins in	Action lasts
Crystalline Zinc	Clear	R	1 hour	4 hrs.
Protamine Zinc	Cloudy	P	4 to 6 hrs.	24 to 32 hrs.
NPH (Isophane)	Cloudy	N	4 hrs.	24 hrs.
Lente	Cloudy	L	1 to 2 hrs.	24 to 32 hrs.
Semilente	Cloudy	S	1 to 2 hrs.	To 12 hrs.
Ultralente	Cloudy	U	6 to 8 hrs.	36 hrs.

The kind of insulin a diabetic takes depends upon the
nature of his ailment and is determined by his physician.
The diabetic's doctor will tell him what kind of insulin
to use, the size of the dose, when and how to inject it,
what precautions to take against the possibilities of dia-

betic acidosis and insulin shock.

Things to Know About Insulin

Very few diabetics have a true allergy to insulin. But during the early weeks of treatment, 10 to 20 percent of the patients using insulin have minor reactions consisting of local itching, swelling or pain. Ordinarily these symptoms vanish by themselves after two or three weeks. If they persist or are more severe, the doctor may prescribe oral antihistamines or he may, in some cases, recommend that an antihistamine be mixed in the syringe with the insulin.

In some cases the diabetic may have an allergy to beef or pork protein. In that event insulin from mixed sources should be avoided. As soon as the nature of the allergy is determined, a special insulin derived from the non-allergy-producing source can be obtained from Eli Lilly and Co., which produces separate insulins from beef pancreas and pork pancreas as well as from mixed sources.

Many diabetics often want to know which company makes which insulins.

Both Eli Lilly & Co. and E. R. Squibb and Sons make all types of insulin.

Here are some other facts about insulin which diabetics should know:

All insulin is made from either beef or pork pancreas, or both. Where required, however, any type of insulin from either pure pork or pure beef can be obtained. These single-component insulins, as we have already mentioned, are particularly important for patients who may be allergic to one of the two components.

Pork insulin is structurally closer to human insulin than that of any other species. Consequently it is less likely to induce the development of insulin resistance or allergy and is therefore used in some patients who require very large doses.

Each vial of insulin has an expiration date. Ordinarily, the insulin will remain active beyond that date but, except in emergencies where no fresh insulin is available, outdated insulin should not be used. *Unopened vials of outdated insulin can be returned to the pharmacist and exchanged, without cost, for a fresh vial.*

One more fact about insulin before we turn to the equipment needed by the diabetic. *Insulin need not be refrigerated.* Refrigeration is required by law when insulin is stored or kept by the pharmacist. Despite this, insulin that is being used keeps perfectly well at average room temperature.

Protamine zinc, Lente, and NPH are less sensitive to temperature changes than regular insulin, and all, including regular, may be kept at room temperature for the period they are being used. Only the reserve supply need be stored in a cool place. *Furthermore, too much cold as well as too much heat can spoil insulin.* This is important to diabetics who have to travel, as we will show in the following chapter.

The Insulin Equipment

The diabetic who uses insulin *must* have certain equipment available at all times. However, with the introduction of disposable syringes and needles, the daily injection of insulin has been considerably simplified, since they are used once and thrown away. The conventional equipment, while perfectly satisfactory, requires sterilization by boiling and storage in alcohol containers. This could pose a problem, particularly when traveling.

The various materials needed by the diabetic are as follows:

1. INSULIN

The type prescribed by his physician in the proper concentration. An extra vial or two should be kept in reserve in a cool place. Every diabetic should also have a vial of regular insulin on hand in the event of some emergency such as the need for extra insulin.

2. SYRINGE

Insulin syringes, either glass or disposable plastic, are available for either U40, U80, or U100 concentrations. The syringes are color-coded: red for U40, green for U80, and black for U100. The syringe used should be matched to the insulin concentration used, since this will prevent errors in dosage. There are even special syringes for blind and physically handicapped diabetics which can be preset to the required dose. In all cases, more than one syringe should be available.

3. HYPODERMIC NEEDLE

The needle should be of rustless or stainless steel, ½ to ⅝ inches long. It should be 25- to 26-gauge. A finer gauge, such as 27, may be used *only* with regular insulin. The other insulins would tend to clog. Twenty-five- to 26-gauge needles, however, can be used with any insulin. As for the type of point, an ordinary beveled point retains its sharpness better than the more expensive Huber point. A reserve supply of needles should always be kept on hand because needles may bend or break and, in any case, usually become dull after about two weeks' use.

4. DISPOSABLE EQUIPMENT

Several types of disposable syringes and needles, as well as complete kits, are now available. The most convenient, and also the most expensive, is the syringe with a fixed needle which is presterilized and should be discarded after one use. This syringe is believed less likely to produce air bubbles when insulin is drawn, and there is no dead space where insulin can be trapped. Somewhat less expensive is the plastic syringe with disposable needles. The syringe may be used for one or two weeks, while the presterilized needles must be discarded after a single use. The Monojet disposable syringe made by Sherwood of St. Louis Missouri, is said to have a smaller gauge needle and may be less painful to use.

These disposable plastic syringes are not available everywhere and, because of their greater expense, are not used under the National Health Plan in Great Britain, for example, which favors the glass syringe and stainless steel needle which can be used over and over for many months but must be sterilized with each use.

5. ALCOHOL AND STERILE COTTON

These are essential for sterilization of the top of the insulin vial which will be punctured by the needle and for the site of the injection. Pure grain ethyl alcohol is *not* essential. Denatured and isopropyl alcohol—ordinary rubbing alcohol—does the job just as well *and is much less expensive.* Disposable, alcohol-impregnated swabs packed in tinfoil now are also available for greater convenience.

6. AMPULES OF GLUCAGON

These should be on hand in the event of insulin shock. Glucagon will raise the blood sugar when it is too low or when too much insulin has been taken. Like insulin, this hormone can be injected by any member of the family in the event the patient cannot do it for himself and is unable to take sweets by mouth to counteract shock.

It is prepared by Eli Lilly and Co. and comes in a vial as a powder which is diluted by liquid in an accompanying vial. The entire amount of the diluted powder is injected for adults, and one-half the amount for children.

7. TESTS FOR URINARY SUGAR

Clinitest and Diastix by Ames, and Tes-Tape by Lilly are available. Since daily urine tests are needed in a great many cases, one of these is essential equipment. These test materials show the amount of sugar with varying degrees of accuracy, with Clinitest and Diastix being the most accurate. Since the color guides vary in the different test materials, it is better to record and report the results in percentage or plus values rather than in colors. For example, with Tes-Tape, yellow indicates a negative result for sugar, while with Clinitest and Diastix the presence of sugar is marked by a yellow to orange color. This could certainly cause confusion if the color results were reported without specific reference to the test used.

8. TESTS FOR URINARY ACETONE

The majority of mild diabetics on diet alone probably will not need such tests. For all other diabetics using insulin or oral drugs, four fairly simple tests are available.—Ketostix, Ketodiastix (which measures both sugar and acetone), Acetest, and Acetone Test Powder. One of these should be kept on hand for emergencies which might require a change in treatment, and in those more extreme cases where acetone tests are important.

9. AN IDENTIFICATION CARD

Every diabetic who takes insulin or oral drugs should

carry a card with his name, address, and phone number as well as those of his physician. The card should also state that he is diabetic and should carry the following request:

"If I am unconscious or behaving abnormally I may be having an insulin reaction.

"If I can swallow, give me sugar, candy, fruit juice or a sweetened drink. If I cannot swallow or do not recover promptly, call a physician or send me to the hospital at once."

Standard cards may be obtained free from any affiliates of the American Diabetes Association; Eli Lilly & Co., 740 S. Alabama St., Indianapolis, Ind. 46206; The Upjohn Co., Kalamazoo, Mich. 49001; Ciba-Geigy Corp., Summit, N.J. 07901; the U.S. Vitamin & Pharmaceutical Corp., 800 Second Ave., New York, N.Y. 10017; E. R. Squibb and Sons, 745 Fifth Ave., New York, N.Y. 10022; or from Chas. Pfizer and Co., 235 E. 42nd St., New York, N.Y. 10017.

These nine pieces of equipment are necessary for the diabetic who takes insulin. They should provide him with all he needs to manage the disease. Many other things are made and sold but, except in special cases, are usually unnecessary and merely succeed in adding expense and clutter to the diabetic's life.

There are, for instance, several automatic injectors for diabetics who are reluctant to push a needle into themselves. These should be avoided unless absolutely necessary because it adds an unnecessary gadget and may contaminate the needle. Hypospray is a very expensive gadget which uses a high pressure spring gun in place of a hypodermic syringe and needle and purports to be painless.

CHAPTER 8

Control with Insulin— the Techniques

There is nothing very complicated about an insulin injection. A patient usually learns how to administer it from the physician or· nurse. Furthermore, the whole process is shown pictorially in various pamphlets which can be obtained free of charge from the American Diabetes Association, Eli Lilly & Co., The Upjohn Co., Chas. Pfizer & Co., U.S. Vitamin & Pharmaceutical Corp., or from E. R. Squibb and Sons.

The following is a step by step procedure for use of the disposable syringe:

1. Remove insulin syringe from sterile wrapper.
2. Draw plunger back to desired dosage indication.
3. Remove needle cap.
4. Shake insulin bottle.
5. Wipe bottle top with alcohol.
6. Insert needle into rubber top.
7. Inject air into bottle.
8. Invert syringe and bottle.
9. Fill syringe with desired insulin dose by withdrawing plunger.
10. Remove needle from bottle.
11. Injections should be made in the arms, legs, or abdomen, with a different site in a different area to be used each time.

12. Unless injecting into the arm, steady skin at injection site with two fingers.
13. Wipe injection site with alcohol.
14. Insert needle quickly, straight, all the way.
15. Inject insulin.
16. Withdraw needle.
17. Replace needle cap.
18. Dispose of syringe.

When disposable equipment is not used, the syringe and needle must be sterilized by boiling in water for about five minutes or by constant immersion in alcohol. When alcohol is used, then the syringe and needle should be sterilized by boiling *at least* once every two weeks. Since hard water tends to cake the syringe and needle, make sure soft water is used. If necessary, use distilled water or a commercial water softener. Hard water can usually be detected by a whitish residue it leaves as it boils away. Be careful to eject any water or alcohol remaining in the syringe.

Make sure the insulin to be used is completely mixed in the vial. Only regular insulin needs no mixing. If a mixture of insulins is made in the syringe, make sure they are *thoroughly* mixed. After making the injection, take the syringe apart and rinse with clear water.

These are the steps in taking an insulin injection. It is important to observe them carefully to avoid contaminating the insulin, as well as the danger of injecting too much or not enough insulin. The process is not at all complicated once it is practiced a few times. Child diabetics, no more than four years of age, have been taught to give themselves their own injections.

Insulin Demands Rigid Eating Schedule

Since various insulins have differing times of action, the diabetic must be careful to adjust his meal schedule to the timing of his injections. A change in type of insulin may require a change in eating time.

Injections should also be made the same time each day. If an injection of long-acting insulin is delayed several hours one day, the extended action into the following day may cause too rapid a drop in blood sugar if the next injection is taken on time.

On the other hand, if there is going to be an expected delay in breakfast due, say, to the partaking of Holy Communion, there should be a 25 percent reduction in the dose of long-acting insulin the day before.

There is one fact a diabetic should keep constantly in mind. If he takes insulin it is absolutely essential for him to keep to a rigidly fixed schedule of eating. Even if he has no other dietary restrictions whatsoever, *he must eat at the proper times imposed by the action of the insulin he takes.*

Meals may not be skipped or delayed. They may not be consolidated.

Certain types of insulin even require that the diabetic take between-meal snacks. NPH and Lente insulins, since they reach a high peak of action in the late afternoon, make a snack *imperative* at 4 P.M. This may be a sandwich or crackers and milk or tea. These insulins also make bedtime snacks permissible, but not necessary.

Protamine zinc insulin, on the other hand, if taken in moderate or large doses *demands* a snack before bedtime and makes permissible a crackers-and-milk snack in the late afternoon.

The absolute need for balance between meals, mealtimes and insulin injections should not be hard to understand.

In order to function normally, every human being needs a certain level of sugar in the blood. If this level of sugar rises too high, we have the symptoms of diabetes;

if it falls too low, our nervous systems and brains cannot function normally and we may even develop symptoms of acidosis.

When a diabetic injects insulin, he must be sure that there will always be just enough carbohydrate in his system for the insulin to act upon without upsetting the normal balance. If he eats too much or too frequently for his insulin dose, excess sugar will accumulate in his system. If he eats too little, misses a meal or eats irregularly, at some time during the day the insulin he has injected will have no free carbohydrate to work on. It will therefore go to work on the normally-needed sugar in the blood, nerve and brain tissue, burning it up and causing a sugar shortage—a condition known as hypoglycemia which, unless it is promptly corrected, results in insulin shock.

Insulin and Physical Activity

In addition to making sure his meals and mealtimes are matched to the action of his insulin injections, the diabetic must also try to keep his physical activity as regular as possible. If he is abnormally active, overexerts himself or misses too much sleep, more than the usual amount of sugar is used up, thus leaving less for the insulin to act upon.

Where the variable physical activity is predictable, the insulin dose can be adjusted in advance. A laborer needs less insulin during the week when his work is burning up much sugar than he does on weekends when his major activity is watching television.

In many cases, modern civilization makes it difficult to know in advance when we will be required to produce a burst of physical activity. A man may have to run to catch a train; a woman may have to do emergency cleaning and shopping because of the arrival of unexpected guests; a child may get into a fight or a game and suddenly overexert himself.

Wherever possible, the diabetic must learn how to meet these emergencies. Where he cannot adjust the insulin dosage, he might find it advisable—when physical over-activity is unavoidable—to protect himself with some rapidly available carbohydrate such as candy, a "coke," fruit or fruit juice.

Under most circumstances, the average diabetic who is alert to changing situations and intelligent about his ailment is able to meet emergencies with little if any trouble.

As a matter of fact, it is absolutely astounding that so many patients can be entrusted with self-administration of so potent a drug as insulin and, despite human error and the daily vicissitudes of life, do so effective a job. It is an utterly unique phenomenon unmatched by anything else in medicine.

With the emphasis on making life as normal as possible, there is no reason why the average diabetic should have any qualms about traveling or taking a vacation—going off on a hunting or fishing trip.

Naturally, he must watch his eating schedule and energy output and keep them in balance with his insulin dosage.

- He must take all his necessary equipment with him and have spares of everything available.

He need *not* buy expensive, insulated kits in which to carry his insulin. He *must* be sure that he neither freezes nor overheats his insulin; and that everything he needs for his injections is readily at hand—not packed away in some luggage compartment.

If he is using a plane, insulin placed with the baggage in an unheated baggage compartment will freeze; therefore, he should carry it on his person. If he is traveling by car, insulin kept in the glove compartment may over-heat in the summer. So the diabetic must be sure he carries his insulin in such a way that extremes of heat and cold are avoided.

The sterile, disposable plastic syringes with needles to be used once and discarded are increasingly popular for travel. These, together with alcohol impregnated swabs and such simple tests as Clinitest, Diastix, or Tes-Tape serve to make travel much easier for the diabetic by reducing the bulk of materials that must be carried.

Testing for Sugar and Acetone

Now we come to another task the insulin-taking dia-betic must perform if he is to enjoy the freedom that comes with self-treatment. He must test his urine for sugar and, under certain circumstances, for acetone which appears when fat is used by the body in place of sugar.

The need for testing depends on the nature of the diabetes. The mild diabetic who does not require insulin need not test his urine except during illness or if he is not feeling up to scratch.

If, under these circumstances, sugar does show up, he should test three times daily for two days. If the sugar persists, he should notify his doctor. The mild diabetes may have become aggravated and a change in treatment may be necessary.

The average adult diabetic taking insulin should test his urine for sugar each morning before breakfast. This is a guide to the adequacy of the insulin dose. If sugar is present, an increase in insulin may be necessary. If the insulin dose remains stable, the diabetic might be able to test for sugar every other day with safety. And he need not test for acetone.

If he starts to lose weight he should test twice daily, before breakfast and before dinner. If there is a sharp rise in sugar before breakfast and before the evening meal, he should also test for acetone and inform his physician by telephone. An increase in insulin may be indicated.

If he feels nausea and vomits, the diabetic should test for both sugar and acetone because either an insulin or carbohydrate shortage may be the cause—and the doctor *must* know which it is.

The juvenile diabetic should test for sugar twice daily, before breakfast and before the evening meal. If the sugar test is markedly positive for two tests, there should be a test for acetone.

During any illness, even if it is a common cold, and whether the patient is adult or juvenile, there should be at least three tests a day to check the adequacy of the insulin dose.

In any case, whether the patient is adult or juvenile, or whatever the nature of the diabetes, if the tests show any change from the normal situation the physician should be telephoned.

It is this self-testing, together with the telephone, that makes treatment by remote control possible and gives the diabetic a far greater amount of freedom than would otherwise be possible.

Of the sugar tests available today, the simplest are *Clinitest* and *Diastix*, marketed by the Ames Co. Inc., and *Tes-Tape*, put out by Eli Lilly & Co. Of these, *Clinitest* and *Diastix* are probably the most accurate in showing the precise amounts of sugar in the urine; *Diastix* and *Tes-Tape* are undoubtedly the most convenient.

Clinitest is a modern simplification of the Benedict test which was the test of choice until recently. The ingredients formerly in Benedict Solution are now combined in a tablet with sodium hydroxide to provide heating action which, in the Benedict test, required boiling water. Five drops of urine are measured into a test tube which comes with the test kit. To this, ten drops of water are added. Then a Clinitest tablet is dropped into the tube. As it dissolves it gives off heat and causes bubbling. When the bubbling stops the liquid has changed color. If it is blue, no sugar is present. If it is green, the amount of sugar is slight, ½ percent. If it is yellow, about 1 percent sugar is present. Orange indicates more than 1 percent. Orange-red shows more than 2 percent.

Diastix is a plastic strip with a small paper square at one end. This square turns color one minute after having been dipped and removed from urine. The color changes resemble those of *Clinitest*, with blue-green being negative and brown, positive.

Tes-Tape is a roll of yellow paper which comes in a container similar to Scotch tape. It is impregnated with a dye and the enzyme glucose oxidase which, in the presence of sugar, reacts and liberates the dye. To use it, tear off about 1½ inches of tape, dip it into a urine specimen and hold it for about a minute. Then compare it with the color chart that comes with the package. If the color of the tape remains yellow, there is no sugar. If it turns blue, about 2 percent sugar is present. *It should be noted that the color reactions are opposite to those of Clinitest.* Expiration dates on the Diastix and Tes-Tape packages should be checked, since outdated materials will not react properly.

The modern tests for acetone in the urine are equally simple. The Ames Company puts out *Ketostix*, an impregnated paper strip, and *Acetest*, which uses a tablet; the Denver Chemical Company has *Acetone Test Powder*.

Put a drop of urine on either the Acetest tablet or on

a pinch of Acetone Test Powder or dip a Ketostix strip into the urine. If their color does not change, no acetone is present. If it turns lavender, some acetone is present. If it turns deep purple, a large amount of acetone is present.

Ketodiastix is a plastic strip with two squares at one end. One of these measures sugar, the other measures acetone.

With these basic tests—and with the equipment to give himself injections—the insulin-taking diabetic is able to handle his ailment more or less by himself and with the minimum of dependence on doctor or hospital visits.

Emergencies do arise occasionally, making the physical presence of a doctor necessary at times other than those of the regular check-up examinations.

Apart from illness, infection, or some change in the course of the diabetes itself, there are the questions of insulin shock and diabetic coma which will be discussed in a later chapter. There is also the complication known as fat atrophy.

Fat atrophy due to insulin is found in about 10 percent of all patients. Normally, we all have a layer of fat under the skin. Where atrophy occurs, this fat disappears in the area where insulin is injected, leaving deep hollows. This may happen at only one injection site; it may happen at all sites.

Children and adult females are most susceptible to this complication. It is rare among men. Among children, it may clear up as they get older. Among adults, fat atrophy may be irreversible at times.

The cause of this condition is unknown and there is no definitive treatment. However, it may help to avoid sensitive sites, to keep changing them, and to use smaller amounts of more highly concentrated insulin, to change the type of insulin, and to add small amounts of soluble cortisone to the insulin. Probably the most effective approach to the problem is to use pork Lente insulin, the purest form available.

Today, the average diabetic who takes insulin can—within the framework of his treatment—live a virtually normal life. He can work, play, marry, become a parent, and do just about anything else that a non-diabetic can do. In short, insulin has made it possible for even the severe diabetic to live with his disease.

CHAPTER 9

The Oral Drugs

While the epoch-making discovery of insulin provided the diabetic with a means of controlling his disease, it also created a whole new set of problems.

To some, injections are painful and unpleasant. To others they are a distinct hardship. Still others find it impossible to inject themselves and must have it done for them—usually by a member of the family or by a friend trained to do the job.

What is more, the insulin-sensitive diabetic faces the hazard of insulin reaction, and even those who are not sensitive must observe a rigid schedule of eating and physical activity.

Almost from the moment insulin was put into use, diabetics and their physicians began to hope for some safe, effective, and inexpensive treatment that could do what insulin did but that need not be injected.

Insulin pills or capsules were out of the question. Almost since its isolation researchers have been trying to find some way insulin could be administered orally. So far, the problem has been insoluble. The reason: Insulin is a protein substance which cannot be swallowed and absorbed into the system without being destroyed by the digestive juices.

So, while a few scientists continued to look for some way to make an insulin that could be taken by mouth, others turned their attention to other possible substances.

The problem was to find something which could be taken by mouth to reduce high blood sugar, help the body metabolize carbohydrates and—at the same time—produce no dangerous reactions. This last requirement proved one of the major obstacles. Drugs were found that could reduce blood sugar, but they also damaged the kidneys, liver or other organs.

Remedies were hunted almost everywhere. Some investigators tried herbs such as mushrooms, carrots, and whortleberry leaves. Some used onion juice, yeast extracts, and microbes from the intestines of birds. Not even the lore of witch doctors was overlooked as "cures" were tried from the jungles of Africa and North Borneo.

In 1926, a group of German scientists headed by Dr. E. Frank, working in the laboratory of Dr. Minkowski in Breslau, announced that they had developed an effective chemical which could be taken by mouth to reduce blood sugar. This was a relative of a substance found in turnip juice and earthworms; and it was named Synthalin.

Synthalin was brought to the market much too rapidly, and, while it appears to have been effective in lowering blood sugar, it produced damage to the liver in more than 40 percent of the patients who used it. The drug was therefore discontinued.

Accident Provides Clue to Oral Drug

The first hint in the 30-year search which ultimately led to an effective oral drug came as the result of a medical accident. A group of French chemists had produced a sulfa drug variation which they thought might be taken by mouth to treat typhoid. In the early part of 1942, they sent it to the Montpellier Clinic for Contagious Diseases in Southern France, where Marcel Janbon began to test it on typhoid patients.

Shortly after the drug was administered, some of the

patients developed unusual symptoms. They began to perspire, became faint and dizzy; they trembled and became disoriented. Two of the patients, a girl of 19 and a woman of 31, died.

Puzzled by these effects, Janbon consulted a brilliant young physiologist at the University of Montpellier, Dr. Auguste Loubatières. Immediately suspecting that the anti-typhoid drug had produced symptoms resembling insulin shock, Loubatières began a series of tests on laboratory animals.

He found that his suspicion had been correct. The sulfa drug, known as 2254-RP, did lower blood sugar. However, it only did this when some part of the pancreas was present and, apparently, some insulin was being produced in the body. Where there were no insulin-producing islets of Langerhans, 2254-RP was ineffective.

Since this particular sulfa drug was not safe for use in humans, Loubatières went to work with a number of related drugs and published a series of papers on the results of his efforts. For some reason, perhaps because of the war and the fact that France had been overwhelmed by the Germans, this path-breaking work by Loubatières was generally overlooked. Scientists, even in the United States, knew about it—yet, incredibly, it was ignored.

Despite this, Loubatières stubbornly continued his work, studying the manner in which various sulfa drugs acted to reduce blood sugar in the body. It was not until Orinase became generally accepted that his vital contributions received belated recognition.

The second step along the path to an oral anti-diabetes drug was almost an exact duplication of the first. This time, the scene was Berlin, and the time was 1954—twelve years after the tests at Montpellier.

Karl Joachim Fuchs, a young resident at the Augusta-Viktoria Hospital in Berlin, received a newly developed sulfa drug from his superior, Hans Franke, and was asked to test its germ-killing possibilities.

It was a fairly routine assignment since many new drugs were constantly being tested. So Fuchs administered it to patients suffering from various infections such as pneumonia and other ailments. This new drug was named BZ-55.

Apparently BZ-55 was an effective germ killer. Many patients showed prompt relief following administration of the drug. But, here and there, Fuchs noted peculiar reactions. Some patients were perspiring violently, shaking, dizzy, and confused. They reacted exactly as though they were approaching a state similar to insulin shock.

So Fuchs decided to try BZ-55 on himself. He swallowed several tablets and watched the developing symptoms of perspiration, faintness, dizziness, trembling, and hunger. A test of his blood sugar showed it had dropped far below normal.

When the results were reported to Franke, an expanded series of tests were begun. Diabetic patients were taken off insulin and given BZ-55 in its place. The drug showed itself effective in about 80 percent of the cases. It brought blood-sugar down to normal and seemed to provide generally good control.

Concurrently, in Hamburg, Germany, Dr. Ferdinand Bertram was trying BZ-55 on a group of diabetic patients at the Barmbek General Hospital. The results were startlingly like those in Berlin.

Juvenile and insulin-deficient diabetics were *not* helped by the drug. But adult-onset diabetics showed amazingly good results.

Reports of the new drug were received with considerable caution in the United States. This was due to a number of factors, among which was the unhappy fact that Synthalin had proved toxic.

Eli Lilly & Co. of Indianapolis brought BZ-55 to the United States and gave it out for testing. In October, 1956, after considerable investigation and trial on human volunteers, the drug was withdrawn. It *was* highly effective, American researchers agreed, but in about five percent of the cases it was said to produce dangerous side reactions. In this respect, American findings disagreed with those in Germany and other European countries where the drug was announced as safe and was put into regular use.

Sugar Control with Minimal Side Effects

BZ-55 is a germ-killing sulfa drug and these drugs are known to have side reactions associated with their antibacterial activity. This brought a focus of interest on a sulfa-related drug which had *no* germ-killing qualities but *did* reduce blood sugar.

This new drug was developed in Germany in 1954 at the laboratories of the Farbwerke Hoechst Company. Called *tolbutamide*, this chemical is a sulfonylurea, related to the sulfas but not a true sulfa itself. It has absolutely no effect upon bacteria and apparently produces none of the side reactions usually connected with its germ-killing cousins.

Doctors in various parts of Germany tested it on more than 780 diabetics in a series of preliminary trials and reported that it was effective in more than half of the cases, producing remarkably slight side reactions.

The possibilities looked so promising that The Upjohn Co. of Kalamazoo, Michigan, brought the drug into the United States and, showing extreme caution, subjected the drug to one of the most careful investigations undergone by any substance in modern medical history.

The drug, known as Rastinon abroad, was given the trade name of Orinase in the United States and Canada.

It was received by Upjohn in November, 1955, and put to preliminary laboratory tests on various animals including dogs, rabbits, chickens, ducks, and frogs. C. J. O'Donovan of Upjohn, who was responsible for evaluating the results of the tests, was interested in first obtaining some standard of reference as to the drug's safety, efficiency, and proper dosage levels.

After these factors were established, a number of outstanding specialists in the field of diabetes were asked to begin preliminary tests on human patients in carefully controlled hospital environments where each reaction could be accurately checked. After about two months of this testing, sufficient data had been collected to permit the start of large-scale tests which began in February, 1956.

By the time tolbutamide was finally released to physicians for general use by the Food and Drug Administration in June, 1957, it had been tested on about 20,000 selected patients. More than 3,000 physicians were involved in these tests, and detailed reports on 7,000 cases were received from 400 physicians and clinics.

The results showed that tolbutamide was *not* an insulin substitute. It was not effective in *every* case where insulin was being used. But, for about half of the diabetics who took insulin, tolbutamide could replace insulin in controlling diabetes.

Where the patients were over 40, tolbutamide was effective in three out of five cases.

Where the patients were between 20 and 40, tolbutamide helped one out of three cases.

In juvenile diabetes and where the patients were under 20, tolbutamide was only occasionally effective.

Clearly, for a large number of diabetics, tolbutamide presaged a revolution in treatment virtually as great as that brought about by the discovery of insulin.

Oral Drugs—Their Mode of Action

The success of tolbutamide led to various modifications of the basic formula in an effort to find more effective forms. Several that were developed failed because of toxicity. Three modifications, however, were put into general use several years after tolbutamide.

One of these is Diabinese, known chemically as chlorpropamide, manufactured by Chas. Pfizer & Co. This is a chlorinated form of the basic sulfonylurea structure. It has increased potency—five to six times greater than that of tolbutamide. But increased potency is achieved at the price of increased side effects, a fact which applies, generally, to all drugs, not just chlorpropamide.

The advantage offered by chlorpropamide's greater potency lies in the fact that a smaller does is required—never more than two pills daily—and its prolonged action makes a single administration a day possible. But the cost is possible jaundice, sodium retention and consequent fluid retention or edema, and—especially in the elderly—the possibility of low blood sugar during the overnight fast.

In 1964, Eli Lilly & Co. introduced Dymelor, chemically called acetohexamide, another form of the basic sulfonylurea. Its potency is intermediate between tolbutamide and chlorpropamide.

Tolinase, chemically called tolazimide, was introduced by Upjohn in 1966, and is more potent than tolbutamide or acetohexamide. All these sulfonylureas act by stimulating an increased release of insulin from the pancreas.

When tolbutamide was first introduced, its mode of action remained a mystery. Research has since shown that these sulfonylureas all act by stimulating an increased release of insulin from the pancreas.

An entirely different oral drug has also been developed

by the U.S. Vitamin & Pharmaceutical Corp. This is known as DBI, or phenformin. DBI is now being distributed by Ciba-Geigy, while U.S. Vitamin distributes the same drug under the name of Meltrol.

Unlike the sulfonylureas, the action of phenformin does not duplicate the effect of insulin but lowers the blood sugar in some manner not yet understood. However, two things are known: it somehow interferes with sugar absorption from the intestine; it enhances breakdown of sugar by a method entirely different from that used by insulin.

Like insulin, the oral drugs are not the perfect answer to diabetes. They are *not* a cure. They are only a form of treatment. They are easier to use than insulin, offer fewer complications, and permit greater freedom of living habits. But, where they can replace insulin therapy in *many* cases, they cannot replace insulin in *all* cases.

For the oral drugs to work, some part of the pancreas must be present and in working order. In no case have they been known to work where the pancreas has been removed or where the islets of Langerhans were destroyed.

Nor are oral drugs indicated in severe diabetes, in juvenile or insulin-deficient diabetes, or in cases where the diabetic is severely ill, undergoing surgery, or suffering acidosis. But, even in these situations, there appear to be some areas where they *do* work. Which further emphasizes that diabetes is a disease—or group of diseases— where a vast amount of exploration remains to be done, and where the exceptions frequently *upset* the rules.

For example, oral drugs are generally not effective in juvenile diabetes according to the results of much valid testing. Yet, a small number of juvenile diabetics have responded favorably to oral therapy. Physicians simply run routine tests to see how patients respond to the new drug and whether they can be changed over. Occasionally, patients who, according to statistics, *cannot* be changed over, make the change with no difficulty. In other cases, patients who should have no trouble at all cannot be changed.

Why or how this should be so is one of the mysteries of diabetes that remains to be explained.

Ordinarily, oral drugs can best replace insulin where the need for insulin is about 40 units or less daily. In some exceptional cases, patients receiving 60 or even 100 units of insulin daily have successfully changed to oral therapy.

Treating the Diabetic with Oral Drugs

Oral drugs either work well or they do not work at all. This fact makes it simple for the physician to determine whether oral therapy is practicable.

Such a decision has to be made whenever a patient is newly diagnosed as diabetic. It may also become necessary with the established diabetic, one who has previously been treated with diet alone or with insulin injections and diet.

Where the patient who is being treated with dietary restriction alone shows failing results in control of the disease, he becomes a candidate for either insulin or oral therapy.

Similarly, the established diabetic who has not been treated at all should be considered for oral treatment.

As for the insulin-treated patient, there are a number of reasons that might make him suitable for one of the oral drugs. The patient might be unwilling or unable to take the injections. He might develop an insulin allergy. For these or other reasons, the physician might decide his patient a proper subject for one of the pills.

Where this is the case, probably the easiest way to effect a change to oral therapy is by a gradual withdrawal of insulin. Parallel with this withdrawal, maximum doses of the oral drug—if it is a sulfonylurea—are administered until the insulin is completely discontinued. If the diabetes remains under control, the dose of sulfonylurea is then gradually reduced to the smallest dose required to maintain this control. However, if there is any sign that the disease is not being controlled, the patient should be returned to insulin at once.

In contrast, patients who have not taken insulin in the past—whether these are newly diagnosed diabetics or individuals who have been treated with diet or received no treatment at all—are given initially small doses of any oral drug. These are then gradually increased until control is achieved.

The maximum maintenance dose for the sulfonylurea drugs would be, generally, six tablets daily of tolbutamide, four tablets daily of acetohexamide or tolazimide, and two tablets daily of chlorpropamide.

Phenformin, which is not a sulfonylurea, is administered somewhat differently from the other drugs. Under no circumstances, even when the patient is being changed over from insulin, are large doses used initially. The rule with this drug seems to be: "Start low, go slow."

The reason for this is the incidence of appetite loss, gas, diarrhea, nausea and vomiting which may develop at the higher dosage levels. Therefore, all diabetics who are given this drug are begun on the lowest possible dose, which is gradually increased to the point where, consistent with drug safety, the diabetes is controlled. Unfortunately, some patients cannot tolerate this drug even at the minimum dose. DBL has a higher risk of toxicity and therefore should be used only after the sulfonylureas and insulin have failed. Because of its severe side effects in a few patients, this drug may be withdrawn.

There are some additional factors to be considered when the newly diagnosed diabetic is introduced to treatment. While such a patient will usually require the smallest dose, this is not always the case.

In exceptional instances, where the symptoms are pro-nounced or severe, the physician might decide it more appropriate to initiate therapy with insulin or the largest dose of sulfonylurea drug in order that control be estab-lished as quickly as possible. In effect, the treatment of any patient—new or old—will reflect the severity of the clinical picture. For this reason, while rules of treat-ment are essential, the therapy should be adjusted to the particular needs of the patient.

For the patient whose diabetes was discovered acci-dentally, perhaps during the course of a general physical examination, and who is free of symptoms, the use of an oral drug will offer several benefits.

It will help maintain control of the diabetes during periods of stress and overeating. In addition, there may be a long-term benefit for the patient in that the oral therapy could have the effect of slowing, or even stop-ping, what would otherwise be an inexorable progression of the disease. These patients may even be prevented from becoming insulin-dependent in later life.

If a patient, previously untreated with insulin, fails to show good results with one oral drug, success is still possible by changing to any one of the others. If each of the drugs fails singly, a combination of any of the sulfonylureas with phenformin might still prove effective.

The diabetic who is being successfully treated with oral medication may, under certain circumstances, have to be changed to insulin temporarily. This may take place during illness or infection; if some unusual stress produces a great metabolic strain; during surgery or, possibly, during pregnancy. In most of these cases, once the situation returns to normal, the patient can resume the oral drug.

However, should the diabetes itself change and as-sume a more severe form, the patient may have to make a permanent change from oral to insulin therapy.

The chart of available oral drugs on page 119 should prove useful for quick reference.

The choice of drug will be made by the physician on the basis of his estimation of the requirements of the disease as well as the needs of the patient.

From the standpoint of safety, tolbutamide has an unparalleled record.

Today, however, there is a drug 100 times more potent than tolbutamide. Called both glybenclamide and glyburide, this drug was developed by Hoechst in Germany and is available under various trade names throughout the world, but *not* in the United States. It is used in very small doses of 5 mg one to three times daily and provides the effectiveness of maximum doses of the other sulfonylureas. Although the amounts required are exceptionally small, glybenclamide's extreme potency may evoke as yet undetermined side effects.

The Oral Drug Controversy

After 13 years of successful clinical use in the United States, a controversy developed around the oral drugs in May, 1970. Following a study which indicated that patients treated by diet alone suffered fewer complications and cardiovascular deaths than those treated with oral drugs and insulin, the Food and Drug Administration presented limits on the advisability of oral drug use in the treatment of diabetes.

There was a feeling that oral drugs and even insulin had been used with decreasing emphasis upon dietary restriction as the foundation of diabetes treatment, and that patients were taking medications unnecessarily in cases where closer adherence to diet could be obtained to control the disease.

The press releases at the time created considerable anxiety and even panic among diabetic patients, particularly those using oral agents.

Data disputing and even contradicting the conclusions of the study on which the Food and Drug Administration action was based came from centers both here and abroad. Moreover, the government agencies regulating drug use in Canada, England, Sweden, and Germany refused to accept the FDA's conclusions and consequently did not impose any limits on the use of oral drugs in the treatment of diabetes.

In the United States the drugs have not been removed from the market, but guidelines for their use have been set up, with the physician being given the responsibility of choosing patients with greater selectivity. Needless to say, many specialists do not agree with the FDA and are continuing to treat their patients as before.

Advantages of Oral Therapy

For the patient who takes an oral drug, life with diabetes is much easier than for the one who needs insulin.

This goes far beyond the obvious fact that it is easier to swallow a tablet than to plunge a hypodermic needle into one's skin every day. Wherever oral drugs work, they seem to provide better control over diabetes than does insulin. They leave the urine sugar-free, significantly reducing the hazard of insulin reaction.

This is most important psychologically as well as physiologically. For the diabetic, it means release from a threat against which he must be on constant guard when taking insulin. He is relieved of the worry as well as the possible damage associated with hypoglycemia.

And, of course, the actual business of living is vastly

simplified by oral therapy. The insulin-treated diabetic, to avoid the possibility of a reaction, must adhere to a rigid eating schedule. If he misses or delays a meal, he faces the risk of hypoglycemia. Similarly, if he overworks or even underworks, he may run into insulin or diabetic complications. None of this seems to be true for the patient who takes an oral drug. Somehow, this drug provides the diabetic with a new dimension of latitude in living.

The advantages of oral drugs extend beyond the realms of convenience and safety from insulin reaction. Many diabetics, because of enfeeblement, advanced age, disease or some disability, are unable to give themselves injections and must have someone else do the job for them. In one case a son had to drive twenty miles every morning to give his mother the insulin injection she could not give herself.

Oral medication, on the other hand, eliminates this problem involving not only the diabetic but the son, the friend, the neighbor, or whoever it is who has to take time off every day to administer the injection.

There are also the matters of employability and insurability, which are affected by insulin. Diabetics who take insulin frequently find that various ordinances may forbid their doing certain work and they may also have greater difficulty in obtaining insurance. Because of the possibility of insulin reaction, they are not permitted to drive public conveyances such as taxis, buses, or trains. But if they take oral drugs this is less of a hazard and they may drive any public conveyance.

Some diabetics who are allergic to sulfa drugs or to antibiotics may hesitate to change to a sulfonylurea through fear of possible allergy reactions. The fact is— and this bears repetition—that while the sulfonylureas are remotely related to the sulfas, they are not true sulfas themselves and do not produce sulfa reactions. Nor are they antibiotics, therefore they do not produce antibiotic side effects.

A further advantage is provided by the oral drug. We know that native insulin, produced in the islets of Langerhans, is carried by the blood directly from the pancreas to the liver, which seems to be its primary site of action. But injected insulin must make its way from the point of injection through the entire circulatory system before even part of it reaches its destination in the liver. On the way, much of it is trapped, blocked, and even destroyed by the action of various body substances.

Obviously, native insulin using the natural pathways to the liver is more effective than injected insulin that must go the long way around. The sulfonylureas, by working through the native insulin mechanism, seem to take advantage of this greater efficiency.

For the diabetic who is now freed from the daily need for an injection, the advantage of an oral drug is immediate and obvious. But the new drugs are having more far-reaching effects by spurring a new wave of diabetes research.

It is in this upsurge of scientific investigation, using them as research tools, that the greatest value of the new drugs may ultimately be found. For instance, experiments into the manner in which they work may provide a clue as to how insulin works. This, in turn, may offer a key to the mystery of diabetes itself—its cause or causes, and perhaps a possible cure.

ORAL HYPOGLYCEMIC DRUGS

Trade Name	Generic Name	Type	Manufacturer	Size of Tablet	Daily Dose	Duration of Action
Orinase	tolbutamide	sulfonyl-urea	Upjohn	.5 gm (500 mg)	1 to 6 tablets (usually twice daily)	6 to 12 hours
Dymelor	acetohexa-mide	sulfonyl-urea	Lilly	.5 gm (500 mg)	1 to 4 tablets (once or twice daily)	12 to 14 hours
Tolinase	tolazimide	sulfonyl-urea	Upjohn	.1 gm (100 mg) .25 gm (250 mg)	100 to 750 mg	12 to 14 hours
Diabinese	chlorpropa-mide	sulfonyl-urea	Pfizer	.1 gm (100 mg) .25 gm (250 mg)	100 to 500 mg daily	to 60 hours
DBI	phenformin	phenethyl-biguanide	Ciba-Geigy	.025 gm (25 mg)	2 to 6 tablets (two or three times daily)	4 to 6 hours
Meltron	phenformin	phenethyl-biguanide	U.S. Vit.	.025 gm (25 mg)	2 to 6 tablets (two or three times daily)	4 to 6 hours
DBI-TD	phenformin	phenethyl-biguanide	Ciba-Geigy	.05 gm (50 mg) per capsule	1 to 2 capsules (once or twice daily)	8 to 12 hours
Mel.-TD	phenformin	phenethyl-biguanide	U.S. Vit.	.05 gm (50 mg) per capsule	1 to 2 capsules (once or twice daily)	8 to 12 hours

CHAPTER 10

The Complications of Diabetes

Today's diabetics, unlike those of half a century ago, can usually manage their disease with relative ease. Were it not for two major complications, they would have little to bother with apart from the ordinary steps involved in treatment. These complications—insulin shock and diabetic coma—do more than disturb the normal tenor of diabetes control. It is through them that diabetes can do its most serious damage.

The patient taking insulin is subject to insulin reaction and shock.

Diabetic coma, a hazard faced by all diabetics who allow the disease to get out of control, is more likely among those who are insulin-deficient.

Of the two complications, insulin reactions, or hypoglycemia (low blood sugar), are more common and more sudden in onset. Diabetic coma is slow in onset and may take 24 hours or more to develop. But insulin reaction can literally happen in an instant. A diabetic may seem perfectly normal one moment, be unconscious the next.

For this reason, if a diabetic is ever uncertain as to whether any abnormal symptoms are due to insulin reaction or the development of coma, he should act at once to block insulin reaction. If he is wrong, he will have time to correct the error.

The Hazard of Insulin Reaction

Insulin reaction or *hypoglycemia*, is the result of too rapid and extreme a drop in blood-sugar. Ordinarily, a normally healthy man has about a teaspoonful of sugar in his blood before breakfast. This rises slightly after each meal but is kept within a normal range by the insulin discharged by his pancreas. *At no time does his pancreas produce more insulin activity than is needed to keep his blood sugar at a normal level.*

A diabetic's blood-sugar level is higher than normal before breakfast and rises more than normally after each meal. Since the normal insulin supply cannot control this he must inject additional insulin. *This injected insulin does not match its activity to the blood-sugar level as does the natural insulin produced in the body.*

Whenever a diabetic has *more* insulin activity than can be matched by the available blood sugar, the excess insulin produces such abnormally low blood-sugar levels that the brain and nervous system are deprived of an essential source of energy. The result is an insulin reaction which, if unchecked, can rapidly lead to shock.

Such a reaction might result from any of a number of situations which cause either too little blood-sugar or too much insulin activity.

A diabetic might miss a meal because of the rush of work; delay a meal to tend a crying baby; fast during a Holy Day or skip a meal in preparation for Communion; become nauseated, vomit, have diarrhea—either from stomach upset, motion sickness, the taking of a purgative or emetic, an emotional upset, or some other cause; engage in unexpected physical activity such as playing some extra holes of golf or doing some hectic shopping in a crowded store.

All of these situations, by reducing the amount of available food or by using it up too swiftly, lower the level of blood sugar which the insulin dose is balanced to match. This brings about a relative excess of insulin and a raid into the body's *needed* store of sugar.

On the other side of this delicate balance, shock can be the product of simply too much insulin.

After many years of daily insulin injections, the process becomes so automatic and unthinking that a diabetic might measure an overdose without being aware of it. He might even forget that he has already taken an injection. Perhaps he was not fully awake or was thinking of something else at the time. So he takes another injection.

In all these cases the food intake and available blood sugar may be exactly as planned. The oversupply of insulin is what causes the trouble.

This about sums up the categories of things that could set the stage for an insulin reaction, but there is one special situation that deserves mention—drinking. For the diabetic, social drinking may sometimes be as perilous as extreme alcoholism.

This *does not* mean that the average adult with diabetes must abstain from alcohol for medical reasons. On the contrary, circumstances exist where alcohol is useful in diabetes. But it *does* mean that the diabetic who takes a drink must be particularly careful not to let his drinking unhinge his sense of time. The drink that makes a diabetic delay a meal is the drink too many. Nor is this the only potential danger.

A business associate invites a diabetic to have a drink after work. The diabetic agrees. He has a drink, then another. Even if he were not diabetic, several drinks would do something to his sense of time. Before he knows it, he has missed his train home and must wait for another.

By late afternoon, his insulin activity is reaching a peak. Maybe, if he is feeling no pain, he decides to have another drink. Maybe not. In any case, whether he realizes it or not, he is missing the meal he should be eating to accommodate the insulin in his system.

He begins to sweat, feels a little dizzy perhaps. It might be the liquor. So he leaves his friend and goes out into the air. Perhaps he decides it is time to try again for the train. Meanwhile the insulin, hungry for sugar, deprives his nervous system and cerebral cortex of this vital energy source.

Suddenly, in the street, he staggers and collapses, struck down by insulin shock. A well-meaning passer-by bends over to help, smells the alcohol on his breath, shrugs and moves on. No point getting mixed up with a drunk.

Because his collapse is mistaken for drunkenness, the underlying insulin shock may be undetected and untreated long enough to cause irreparable damage.

Even without the smell of liquor on a diabetic's breath, the symptoms of insulin reaction often look enough like drunkenness to make a mistake all too easy. This makes it more important for the diabetic to carry a card, easily accessible, identifying him as a diabetic and describing what to do in emergencies.

He should also let his friends, neighbors, associates, classmates, and teachers know he is diabetic. Diabetics, especially adolescent girls and young women, frequently try to keep their ailment a secret, thus adding to their own difficulties in an emergency.

Finally, the diabetic—as well as those associated with him—should know the symptoms of insulin reaction and be able to recognize them promptly and treat them.

How to Recognize and Correct Insulin Reaction

The first sign of an insulin reaction is usually mild hunger. Then, in order, come

> sweating
> dizziness
> hunger
> palpitation
> pale, moist skin

If the reaction is untreated, these symptoms follow:

> trembling
> blurred or double vision
> mental confusion and disorientation
> very strange behavior (disrobing or something equally odd)
> finally, the end symptom, loss of consciousness

At any point before unconsciousness sets in, taking a lump of sugar, a piece of candy, drinking soda pop, fruit juice or anything else containing sugar can abolish the symptoms swiftly.

There is hardly anything in all of medicine as dramatic as the almost instantaneous correction of insulin reaction after the administration of sugar. That is why the diabetic on insulin should always carry an emergency supply of hard candy or lump sugar. Within minutes after the sugar is swallowed there usually is a complete return to normality with, oddly enough, no memory of what took place after the start of mental confusion.

Recovery is not so prompt for the diabetic whose insulin reaction is untreated until he is already unconscious. In that case it may be 15 minutes before recovery becomes apparent, and the diabetic may be left with a headache.

If left untreated for too long, the reaction may be so severe that the diabetic cannot swallow candy or sugar.

In that case, a doctor should be called at once. He should also be called if the patient does not respond to treatment.

If possible, glucagon should be administered by hypodermic as an emergency measure. Glucagon ampoules are part of the necessary equipment for all insulin-sensitive diabetics. The doctor, when he arrives, will probably administer glucose in order to raise the blood sugar with the least possible delay.

The longer the patient is unconscious before treatment begins, the slower and less complete will be the recovery.

It is important for every diabetic and everyone close to him to remember that repeated and prolonged incidents of insulin reaction can have cumulative effects. Therefore, they must be avoided or, if they do occur, treated the instant they are *suspected*. The diabetic who feels a growing hunger or thinks he is perspiring should never wait to see if the symptoms will go away by themselves—no matter how mild they seem.

The *first suspicion*, however slight, should be treated without delay as a full onset of insulin reaction. Where insulin reaction is concerned, the diabetic must take absolutely no chances. It is far better to take emergency sugar unnecessarily than to risk shock.

There is a wide variety of sugars and sweets that can help a diabetic overcome insulin reaction. These include sugar, fruit juices, sweetened drinks, syrups, soda pop, honey, jams and jellies, candies.

Artificial sweeteners and sugar substitutes are absolutely useless and must *never* be used in these cases. This applies to the so-called diabetic candies, jellies, jams, and similar products. These may be fine in the ordinary diabetic diet where sugar is being avoided. But in the event of an insulin reaction *real* sugar is essential.

Whole fresh fruit, bread, or other starches are of no

immediate value, since they are too slowly digested to compensate for an acute sugar shortage. The diabetic in shock should not be given too much sugar too rapidly or he may become nauseated.

It is better to administer a lump of sugar or a glass of fruit juice. Then, as his mental powers recover, give him a bit more. The important thing is the speed with which the sugar is given, not the amount. After the patient has emerged from the reaction, he should be given some regular nourishment—fruit, bread, or other high-carbo-hydrate food—to provide a reserve of sugar for later use.

Before leaving the subject of insulin reaction, it would be wise to emphasize once more the importance of recognizing and treating this condition at once. If a diabetic feels poorly in any way or behaves strangely, *he should be treated for insulin reaction immediately—even if the symptoms are doubtful or do not follow a regular pattern.*

Relatives, friends, and others who are close to the diabetic should be ready to act the instant he shows any deviation from normal behavior.

The teacher should be careful to note inattention on the part of the normally attentive diabetic student.

The wife or associate should suspect that a rise of ir-ritability or temper is a sign of insulin reaction rather than real anger.

The Hazard of Diabetic Coma

Coma, the second major complication of diabetes, is the exact opposite of insulin shock. Shock begins with an abnormal drop in blood sugar due to *too much insulin activity*. Coma develops from an abnormal rise in blood sugar due to *too little insulin activity*.

The development of coma follows the same pattern as

untreated diabetes. Lacking insulin activity with which to metabolize sugar, the body hungrily raids its own fat and protein tissue for substitute energy sources. This brings about a rise of ketone and acetone in the blood; then, as the normally alkaline blood becomes loaded with these fatty acids, acidosis and coma follow.

Unlike insulin reaction, diabetic coma is slow and undramatic in its onset. It is also relatively infrequent today. Yet before the discovery of insulin, many adult and practically all juvenile diabetics eventually died in coma.

The symptoms of diabetic coma are indentical with those of severe diabetes:

> Frequent, copious urination
> Constant thirst
> Flushed, dry skin
> Weakness, fatigue and drowsiness
> Fruity odor of breath
> Deep, labored breathing
> Vomiting
> And finally, unconsciousness

The events leading to coma can be set into motion by any of a wide variety of events.

A patient might be taking drugs which raise the level of blood sugar, such as cortisone or its derivatives, or certain diuretics which are commonly used to rid the body of excess fluids.

An insulin-treated patient may neglect or delay his injections.

A patient using oral drugs may forget to take the tablets.

There might be errors of insulin administration.

A diabetic might use a syringe with the wrong markings and thus take too little insulin.

He might use insulin that is too old or has been spoiled by freezing or overheating.

He might not mix properly an insulin vial that requires mixing—Protamine Zinc, NPH, or Lente.

He might even become involved in something that absorbs his attention and, because insulin injections become unthinkingly routine, imagine that he took it when actually he had not.

These and similar lapses in diabetes control are *external* factors which may precipitate coma by providing less insulin activity than the diabetic normally needs.

There are also *internal* factors that may increase the diabetic's need for insulin above that provided by the usual dose. This can happen in a number of ways—some subtle, some obvious.

As a diabetic grows older he needs less food. If he does not reduce his food intake to match his reduced need, then he will require more insulin. Even if his diabetes had been mild enough to be controlled by diet alone, this may change the nature of his ailment so that a need for insulin develops.

Illness, injury, a decline in physical activity, and various other situations that arise in the course of daily living may result in an increased need for insulin. If unsatisfied, the process leading to diabetic coma is set into motion.

A diabetic catches cold and goes to bed. Because of the decline in physical activity he may need 10 to 12 percent more insulin to handle the sugar which would otherwise have been used up by work, exercise or getting about. If he does not take the extra insulin, in about 24 hours he may have high blood sugar; and the symptoms of diabetes will begin to show themselves almost as though the disease were untreated. Ketosis will follow, then acidosis and, finally, coma. But all this will develop gradually, and with the cushion of time providing a safety factor, the situation should be recognized and corrected before any damage is done.

Just as diabetic coma takes longer to develop than insulin shock, so the response to treatment is equally slow. Insulin reactions are reversed in a matter of seconds when sugar is administered. The trend to coma may take hours to rectify.

Factors That Influence Coma

Gradual though the onset of coma may be, the rate at which it develops is variable, with three factors influencing the tempo.

First, there is the age of the patient. The process is faster in children because they have less sugar stored in the liver than adults and their metabolic needs for growth and energy are higher. Therefore, the raiding of body fat and protein proceeds at a more rapid pace than in adults. In children, the whole process from original insulin deficiency through ketosis, acidosis, and on to actual coma may speed up and take only a day.

Second, there is the nature of the provocation. A cold will not have the same impact on insulin need as will pneumonia. A minor cut will not be as provocative as a multiple fracture. An error in dose will not be as important as failing to take insulin altogether.

Finally, there is the nature of the diabetes. An insulin-deficient diabetic is obviously more susceptible to coma than a maturity-onset diabetic who does produce some natural insulin and is not as dependent upon an outside source. In the latter, internal stress is not as catastrophic and the possibility of an insulin shortage not so serious.

From this standpoint, an attack of lobar pneumonia might be more serious for a young adult diabetic than for an older diabetic. The young adult, with a higher insulin need, would develop ketosis relatively easily. The older diabetic with a slight insulin need, or treating his disease with oral drugs or diet, would have no great problem and might not go into ketosis at all.

Nevertheless, the stress of illness or injury so disturbs the balance of the body that the diabetic who normally can control his disease with only diet or oral therapy may develop a need for insulin during the course of the disturbance. When the provocation is removed, he may return to his usual treatment. All this, of course, is carefully controlled by the physician.

Treatment of Coma

In its early stages, the onset of diabetic coma may be treated at home unless it is complicated by other factors that require hospitalization. The mild-to-moderate ketosis with which the trend to coma begins can be recognized by the symptoms of excessive thirst, frequent urination and a feeling of being "not quite right."

As soon as these symptoms appear the diabetic should rest and avoid any physical activity.

He should test his urine for sugar and acetone.

He should report to his doctor by telephone and, thereafter until the situation is cleared up, should test every urine voided for both sugar and acetone.

If his urine test shows sugar and acetone, he should immediately take an injection of quick-acting regular insulin. In severe diabetes the dose should be 30 to 40 units; in milder cases, 15 to 20 units.

If the urine test shows acetone but no sugar, the diabetic must take candy, honey, sugar, or a sweet drink as well as the insulin injection. This is more common among juvenile diabetics with a low sugar reserve than among adults. The purpose of the sugar is to provide a buffer against the possibility of insulin reaction and to furnish glucose instead of fat as an energy source.

In any case, the diabetic in ketosis should also drink a glass of fruit juice or tea sweetened with 3 teaspoons of sugar every one or two hours.

The same dose of regular insulin should be repeated every two or three hours until the urine is free of acetone. At this time the fruit juice or sweetened drinks may be discontinued and the normal meal schedule resumed.

If the urine tests show high sugar levels even though there is no acetone present; or if the original symptoms persist despite the disappearance of acetone from the urine, the injections of regular insulin should continue at the same intervals, but with only half the original dose. They should be stopped only when the patient feels normal again and his urine is free of sugar.

If the ketosis symptoms are more severe than those mentioned above; should extreme nausea, vomiting, drowsiness, or deep, labored breathing occur, then hospital treatment is probably needed. In any case, the physician should be notified at once.

Although both of the major complications of diabetes arise from opposite causes and require different treatments, they are sometimes confused with one another. For this reason, we will compare their characteristics and show how they can be told apart.

Insulin Reaction	*Diabetic Coma*
Sudden onset	Slow, gradual onset
Perspiration, pale skin	Dry, hot skin
Dizziness	No dizziness
Palpitation	No palpitation
Marked hunger	Little hunger
Normal urination	Excessive urination
Normal breathing	Excessive thirst
Shallow breathing	Deep, labored breathing
Normal breath odor	Fruity breath odor
Confusion, disorientation, strange behavior	Drowsiness and great lethargy leading to stupor
Urinary sugar usually absent or slight, but there may be high sugar left over from hours earlier	Large amounts of urinary sugar
Usually no acetone in urine	Acetone present in urine

By checking these symptoms, it should be fairly easy to distinguish between insulin reaction and diabetic coma. But, if there is any doubt at all, the diabetic should be treated for insulin reaction until a fuller diagnosis is available. The speed of insulin reaction allows no time for delay or error. The slowness of diabetic coma, on the other hand, does grant time for the correction of an error.

Whatever the complication, the physician should be notified at once. The fact that an insulin reaction may be quickly corrected by swallowing a piece of candy, or that ketosis might be eliminated by an injection of regular insulin in no way removes the possibility of danger. The underlying reason for the complication remains to be determined and corrected. That task belongs to the physician.

By curbing the major complications of diabetes—reducing their incidence and correcting them promptly when they do appear—the diabetic may be better able to cope with other ailments which often accompany the disease.

The most common of these is arteriosclerosis or hardening of the arteries. This is a common companion of aging even among non-diabetics, but it frequently appears somewhat earlier in diabetics.

Exactly why certain processes linked with aging should speed up with diabetes is not yet known. Nor does this situation seem to be affected by the quality of diabetes management. Nevertheless, the patient's ability to meet the stresses and strains of daily living as well as the wear and tear of aging can only be enhanced by intelligent care and good control.

What Is Good Control of Diabetes?

The question of what constitutes good control of diabetes is, to put it mildly, open to some discussion. Perhaps "argument" would be a better word to describe the disagreement between the school of the sugar-free urine and the school which disregards urinary sugar.

The best control of diabetes, obviously, would be that which permits the diabetic to live as normally as possible with the greatest protection from complications. There is little question that the reduction of elevated blood sugar levels is crucial. Japanese studies have shown a better degree of reduction of basement membrane abnormalities on kidney biopsy in well-controlled patients than in those who are poorly controlled. Similar observations have been reported from other studies.

Unfortunately, present methods of treatment do not permit blood sugar control to the point where it resembles natural control in the normal person, with subtle mechanisms maintaining a constant balance in accord with the body's needs.

Rigid insistence on sugar-free urine, while it may protect the diabetic from coma, does expose him to a lowered sugar reserve and possible insulin reaction. Child diabetics, whose sugar reserves are naturally low and whose insulin-sugar balance is subject to unpredictable change, cannot maintain a sugar-free urine without teetering on the brink of insulin reaction.

On the other hand, where a sugar-free urine poses no great danger—as in moderate, stable diabetes—the diabetic who has no sugar in the urine *feels better* than one who has some sugar. And the more sugar there is present, the less well he feels. Furthermore, the presence of *unnecessary* sugar may bring the diabetic too close to the slope leading to ketosis, acidosis, and coma.

For these reasons, best control is probably achieved when the following criteria are met:

The diabetic feels well.

His diet permits him to maintain normal weight and provides all the nutritional requirements for growth, work, play, and the regular activities of daily living.

Just enough treatment, whether it be insulin, oral therapy, or dietary restriction, is used to assure proper utilization of the foods eaten without provoking insulin reaction or coma.

The treatment is simplified to the point where the diabetic can live and work with the absolute minimum of interference from the needs of the ailment.

Wherever possible, the diabetic tries to maintain a sugar-free urine or one with the smallest possible amount of sugar.

For about 20 percent of all diabetics—those who are sensitive to insulin and whose disease is unstable, sugar-free urine is impossible. In those cases, moderate amounts of urinary sugar cannot be avoided without running the risk of insulin reaction.

Where these criteria of treatment are met, and there is sufficient flexibility to adjust to whatever changes may occur, then the diabetic has his disease under good control.

Steering a course between excess and insufficient insulin activity, he should then be able to reduce the danger of complications to an absolute minimum while feeling well, working well and living well.

Short of eliminating the diabetes entirely, this is the substantial best that any treatment can seek to accomplish.

PART THREE

The Problems
of Diabetes

CHAPTER 11

The Diabetic Child

It is said that when a child develops diabetes the doctor immediately has two patients—the child and the mother.

This is an understatement.

The diagnosis of diabetes in a child frequently sends out waves of stress which reach far beyond the immediate family.

Not only are the child and mother affected, but so are the father, the other children, in-laws and relatives, friends, and sometimes even teachers. And all these, by their reactions, in turn may affect the child and his attitude toward the disease.

Diabetes in a child is fraught with emotion for the parents and is difficult for them to accept with equanimity. Since there is a possibility of heredity factors being involved, unconscious guilt may assail them. Some even take the attitude that this is a punishment visited upon them from above. Furthermore, the day-in, day-out routine of urine tests, injections, and special eating schedules are chores which the mother must perform; and they are no easy matter to cope with at first.

The mother may react by rejecting the child and treating him with harsh rigidity. She may do the exact opposite and become doting, overprotective, and indulgent. In either case, the child's adjustment to the disease is bound to suffer.

Relatives, especially grandparents, can be very harmful to a child's morale if their reactions are tinged with overanxiety and hysteria. The best intentions of the physician are often thwarted by these attitudes of parents, grandparents and other relatives.

Teachers may be overly disturbed by a child's diabetes and treat him with marked difference from the other children. This is bound to impede the child.

Finally, if there are other children in the family, they are likely to be affected by the situation and, in turn, produce an effect. Depending upon their own security and adjustment, they may tend to resent the special attention given to the diabetic child. The patient, on his part, could easily come to resent the fact that he is suffering the pain of injection and the deprivation of certain foods while the other children are not.

In the face of this downpour of problems, how is the diabetic child ever to achieve proper adjustment to a disease with which he must live the rest of his days? There is no easy, precisely defined answer to this question.

Yet there *is* an answer—one that can be found only in the love and intuitive understanding of the parents.

No normal parents can be expected to accept diabetes in a child casually. But, if they are to help the child, they should place the emphasis on the child rather than on the disease.

This means that they should first accept the child as a human being. The fact that this is a child with diabetes —as it may be a child with any other ailment—is of secondary importance.

The parents should also try to provide a home atmosphere that is relaxed and tranquil, one in which the father as well as the mother plays a positive role. The father's participation in the activities and thought of the child is particularly important and will help provide an additional measure of stability and security. All this will fortify the child, help him withstand the misunderstandings and blunders of overanxious, hysterical, or uninformed outsiders.

How Parents Can Help Diabetic Child

Apart from these general rules, there are some specific suggestions which will help parents—and the child—to achieve a better adjustment to the disease: The parents should become intelligently informed about diabetes; disregard the mysticism, mumbo-jumbo and old-wives' tales and seek out the latest scientific information. They should avoid being either overrestrictive or overindulgent. They should avoid bribery, cajolery, or intimidation to make the child accept injections and other necessities of treatment. They should accept the fact, and try to have the child accept the fact, that the injections, while painful, are necessary. The same applies to such deprivations as denial of certain foods and activities. They should try to treat the disease in such a way that it *seems* to cause the least visible disruption in everyday living. The regular living habits of the family should go on as before. The other children should be treated exactly the same as before, allowed to eat the same, play the same, have the same rights.

By following these suggestions it should be possible for the parents to establish a situation in which the diabetic child has a maximum feeling of security as an individual and as a member of the family. The closer this ideal is approached, the better will be the child's attitude toward his disease; and the fewer will be the strains set up within the family.

The nature of "juvenile diabetes" has already been discussed in the chapter, The Development of Diabetes.

As we know, it erupts dramatically and is usually associated with one or more of the infections so common in childhood. Most often, the child diabetic is already suffering from acute acidosis when the diabetes is recognized, and requires immediate hospitalization. For any child this will be a traumatic experience, but the stronger his sense of security, the better he usually weathers it.

Diabetes Is Bewildering Experience for Child

When the child leaves the hospital and returns home, the whole world seems topsy-turvy. The disease is incomprehensible to him and the attitude he develops will be determined by the attitude and behavior of his parents.

He will discover that he must have at least one injection of insulin a day.

He must have his urine tested for sugar and acetone twice each day, before breakfast and before the evening meal.

He must eat six times a day—three meals and three snacks—at prescribed times and with clock-sure regularity.

His diet is no longer subject to his whim as before—he cannot normally eat sugar, candy, syrups, and soda pop —although he must eat enough of the properly balanced foods to provide for proper growth.

It might be wise here for parents to understand that rapidly absorbed sugars, such as candy, pop, and the like, cause a sharp rise in blood-sugar levels, and a dumping of sugar into the urine whereby it is passed out of the body. This represents wasted eating. On the other hand, these same rapidly absorbed sugars can be very useful in checking insulin reaction where a rapid rise in blood sugar is needed.

The child diabetic, in addition to injections, urine tests

and a rigidly timed eating schedule, must also face certain restrictions on his physical activity. If his insulin action reaches a peak at 3 o'clock, his mother may no longer allow him out in the street to play with the other children at that time, unless he has a snack first. She knows, although he will not, that peak insulin activity coinciding with violent physical activity can result in an insulin reaction.

These changes and restrictions in his mode of life will be beyond the understanding of the young diabetic child. The whole idea of diabetes will be almost impossible for him to grasp, no matter how diligently the parents try to explain. Nevertheless, the young child will usually accept the injections, tests, and restrictions as part of the incomprehensible, inconvenient, and often painful rule imposed on him by the adult world. It is only as he grows older and approaches adolescence that he will begin to question. When this happens, a new set of problems will arise.

Odd Characteristics of Childhood Diabetes

Childhood diabetes has some peculiar characteristics for which the parents should be well prepared.

The first of these can be truly shocking.

About two months or so after the child's disease is diagnosed and treatment begun, there is frequently a dramatic improvement. The symptoms of the disease vanish, the insulin has to be discontinued and the child seems miraculously cured—almost as though the parents' prayers have been answered.

Unfortunately, this is a caprice of the disease. Parents should recognize it as just that, rather than let their hopes be raised, then dashed as the diabetes flares up again permanently, which it inevitably does.

There is another characteristic of childhood diabetes

against which parents should be on guard. Up until about the age of ten, an insulin reaction is often accompanied by symptoms usually associated with the opposite complication—acidosis. These symptoms are vomiting and headache.

Unless the parents are aware of this quirk of the disease and *treat immediately for insulin reaction*, serious error is likely to result.

Even where acidosis *is* the complication involved, *the child who vomits will need sugar along with insulin.*

Treating the Diabetic Child

Ordinarily, the problems of the pre-school diabetic are relatively few, since he is prone to accept parental authority and his environment is more amenable to control. It is easier for a mother to watch over the physical activity and mealtimes of a pre-school child than of a child who spends a large part of the time away from home.

At this stage, the treatment is mainly administered by the parent, who does the testing, gives the injections, regulates eating and, to a lesser degree, physical activity.

Good treatment for a diabetic child generally consists of an adequate diet that permits full growth and enough insulin so that the child can utilize most of the food eaten. Except for the restrictions on concentrated sugars, the diabetic child's diet should be the same in calories and nutrients as that of any normal child his age.

Because of the diabetic child's high sensitivity to insulin, a sugar-free urine may lead to frequent incidents of insulin reaction. So some urinary sugar is permissible at various times during the day. If the morning test shows *no* sign of urinary acetone, control of the child's diabetes is usually good if the child is also growing properly.

Should the child wet the bed, have to urinate frequently or become excessively thirsty, he probably needs a larger dose of long-acting insulin or an extra dose of insulin at night.

The administration of insulin may be one of the most important problems at the outset. There is pain involved and the appearance of the hypodermic syringe is not particularly reassuring. So the child might become frightened and resist the injection.

The parent should try to keep the injection simple and uncomplicated. The syringe should be prepared and the dose measured out of the young child's sight at first. Then the injection should be given with as little fuss as possible.

If the child feels extreme pain, the injections might best be given in the buttocks, which are less sensitive to pain. In extreme cases, the child's resistance might be so great that he will have to be held in order to receive the injection.

Some parents make the mistake of bribing or cajoling the child into accepting the injection. This spoils the child, creates a situation in which he can use the injection as a means of blackmail. Other parents may threaten or scold if the child resists the injection. This will only make him less cooperative later on.

If the child has a normally good adjustment and is accepted, and if the parents are intelligent and understanding, the chances are that the injection will not create too great a problem.

Still, generalizations are always dangerous, particularly so in diabetes. Where injection difficulties arise, the parents should try to ease the situation, keeping one fact firmly in mind: *Whatever the circumstance, the insulin injection must be given in the proper dosage at the proper time.*

In order to prevent the development of problems later in the child's life, it is important for the parent not to be overprotective. As soon as possible, depending upon the age, character and intelligence of the child, there should be a gradual shifting of responsibility for the management of the disease.

Teaching the Child to Treat Himself

The average diabetic child of five can and should be taught to test his own urine for sugar and acetone. This might be done easily by pretending that it is a sort of game. No reading or calculations are involved, only a simple procedure and the matching of colors.

Gradually, after the child has come to accept the injection, the parent can change the sites to include the arms and thighs so the child can see how it is done and, as he develops the ability, be encouraged to do it himself.

By the time the child is eight or nine, he should be taught how to measure his own insulin, prepare and sterilize the syringe.

At about twelve or thirteen, the child ought to be able to take over full responsibility for the management of the disease. He should handle his tests, his injections, watch his diet and activity schedule, be able to detect and control such complications as insulin reaction and acidosis.

Probably the most serious problem of childhood diabetes is the recognition of these complications. The young child is frequently unable to recognize the warning signs of insulin reaction or acidosis. During the excitement of a game, even a passive one, he may disregard the fact that he is perspiring. On the other extreme, he may be too absorbed in other matters to relate the fact that he is urinating frequently.

Sometimes an intelligent child may devise his own approach to the detection of complications. One bright boy of five was able to recognize what he called "a shaky, funny feeling." Whenever he had that feeling he knew he had to take something sweet—usually some candy he carried for such an emergency—and come home for a snack.

Until the child is old enough to detect the symptoms of complications—and even afterwards—the parents, teachers, friends and playmates should be alert for such signs as excessive perspiration, trembling, inattention, irritation or temper in the case of insulin reaction; unusual thirst, frequent urination, weakness or lethargy in the case of acidosis.

Frequently, complications may set in while the child is asleep. For this reason, a parent should, from time to time, pass a hand over the sleeping child's forehead for any sign of perspiration that cannot be attributed to humidity or temperature. A clammy forehead would indicate an insulin reaction, and the child should be given fruit juice or a piece of candy.

On the other hand, a hot, dry forehead, bedwetting or frequent nocturnal trips to the toilet warn of impending ketosis and the need for an injection of 5 or 10 units of regular insulin *plus the feeding of something sweet such as fruit juice.*

Problems of Childhood Diabetes

Because of the extreme instability of juvenile diabetes, many seemingly ordinary things such as season of the year, weather and temperature, may create problems affecting the child's need for insulin. Playing out of doors on a bright, sunny day may reduce his need for insulin. If heavy rains keep him indoors, his physical activity is reduced, causing an increase in insulin need.

When the season and weather permit more physical activity, less insulin is usually needed. Where there is less physical activity more insulin is needed.

In some of the special camps for diabetic children, during rainy weather the children exercise indoors on treadmills to obtain the physical activity they would otherwise miss.

Diabetes does not create serious social problems for the pre-school child. But once the child leaves the shelter of the home to begin his formal education, social as well as new physical problems appear.

The first of these involves integrating the classroom schedule with the child's eating habits. This should not create too great a difficulty if the parents understand that the child's insulin doses and meal schedule may be manipulated to provide an individual adjustment to any new situation.

The type or dose of insulin may be changed to fit the child's new eating program. Similarly, the child's food schedule may be altered to match the insulin activity.

Many children usually need a small dose of quick-acting regular insulin along with a larger dose of slower, long-acting insulin (NPH, Lente, etc.). The regular insulin acts only in the four hours between breakfast and lunch. The long-acting insulin works for the rest of the day.

If the school schedule delays the child's lunch, a reduction in the regular insulin may be necessary to avoid the possibility of insulin reaction. Regular insulin should also be reduced if the child has frequent insulin reactions between breakfast and lunch. On the other hand, if he spills sugar or urinates frequently during that period, regular insulin should be increased.

Similarly, eating schedules can also be modified to meet the needs of living. A child who normally takes the midday meal at 12:00 registers for kindergarten and has to start school at noon. This makes it necessary for him to have the noon meal earlier, say at 11:00, so that he can get to school on time. Since this would mean a longer period without food in the early afternoon and a resulting drop in blood sugar, the child may compensate with a heavier than normal snack at his 3 o'clock eating time.

Strange problems often arise. One particularly bright student who was especially good in arithmetic started a new term by going into an arithmetic slump. His marks were high in every subject but, for some reason, he could not seem to get anywhere with arithmetic.

His doctor heard about it during a routine examination, became suspicious and questioned the boy closely. It turned out that the boy's schedule for the new term was so set up that he had his arithmetic class just before lunch and right after the gymnasium period.

The spurt of physical activity in gymnasium depleted his carbohydrate reserve. When he went into his arithmetic class he was on the threshold of insulin reaction and simply could not concentrate. Then he went to lunch, restored his carbohydrate and finished the rest of the school day with his normal intelligence at full power.

Once the cause for the arithmetic slump was discovered it was easy to correct. A sweet snack at the end of the gymnasium period restored his blood-sugar; and his arithmetic marks rose accordingly.

As the growing child moves out of the home, special alertness is needed to recognize situations of potential conflict between the needs of the diabetes and the requirements of the environment. One way or another, it should be possible to make some sort of accommodation so that the child will be able to function as normally as possible.

Lunches are a common problem for diabetic children. If they eat in the school cafeterias they are usually fed high-carbohydrate meals. While normally quite nourishing, these represent a certain amount of wasted eating for the child who cannot utilize certain carbohydrates as well as other children. For this reason he would be better nourished if he brought his lunch from home—food high in proteins such as meats, fish, eggs, or cheeses, which he can use without waste.

As the child gets older, changes in living patterns bring inevitable changes in the problems of treatment. The child begins to go to bed later, he stays out and plays longer. These and similar developments are bound to demand changes and adjustments in the insulin as well as in the eating schedule.

It is when the diabetic child starts going to school that he will—if he hasn't before—begin to feel the faint stirring of social problems; a realization that he is somehow different from the other children.

During the lunch recess, his classmates may cluster around the "Good Humor" man outside and soon they will all be eating ice cream. All, that is, but the diabetic child. He, for reasons he is probably unable to understand fully, will have to exercise self-discipline and refuse to share in the fun. Not that he can't have ice cream. He can —but only at certain stipulated times within his schedule. But the other children can have their ice cream any time —and as often as they like.

In childhood there is also the flood of birthday parties, becoming more numerous as the child's circle of friends expands. At these parties there is the usual gorging of ice cream, chocolates, layer cake, and other goodies washed down by various kinds of soda pop. The children have a wonderful time stuffing themselves—all but the child diabetic. Such deprivation is usually unnecessary.

If the timing of the party happens to coincide with the child's snack time, the mother should allow the child to have ice cream or cookies. This may help to ease the situation, but it will not entirely remove the mounting sense of "difference."

It is at this stage that the child's feeling of acceptance within the family begins to assume great importance in the diabetes picture. Sparks of rebellion and noncooperation are bound to show as he approaches adolescence. But whether they burst hotly into flame will be greatly influenced by the child's attitude toward his parents—and their attitude toward him.

Both overindulgence and neglect, while they do their damage to the child, are rooted in the personality and adjustment problems of the parents. To correct them, intelligence and human understanding are more important than medical understanding.

But rigid restriction of a child often *can* be corrected by improved medical understanding.

Outmoded Beliefs May Endanger Child

Many doctors, practicing today, retain a number of the old-fashioned attitudes about diabetes. Some even cling to the conviction that diabetes can best be treated by deprivation. These attitudes are passed along to the parents as medical gospel. A situation of rigid control is created, and the child is ultimately bound to rebel, sometimes at considerable damage to himself.

What is more, rigid control is *not* the best control, since it usually increases the incidence of insulin reactions. Children who are allowed only three precisely measured meals a day without extra snacks to compensate for peaks of physical activity are bound to have insulin reactions. Any attempt to correct this situation by decreasing the insulin dose rather than by increasing the flexibility of the food allowance adds a new set of dangers, since the child's insulin needs must invariably grow as he grows.

It is up to the parents to exercise intelligence. They must learn where to establish a balance between the actual needs imposed by the disease and the needs of the child as a human being. They must also be able to draw a line between practices established by medical knowledge and dogmas handed down by custom.

Some parents still believe that everything sweet is dangerous and do not allow their children ice cream or other sweets which *are* permissible, say, as a three-o'clock snack.

In recent years, life for the diabetic child, as well as for the diabetic adult, has eased considerably as far as certain sweets are concerned. Sugar-free "diabetic" ice cream is readily available in most stores, as are many artificially sweetened fruits, cakes, candies, and other foods. Even a sugar-free chewing gum is now on sale. Thus, there is little reason for today's diabetic child to feel a sense of deprivation in this regard. If artificially sweetened desserts and soft drinks are taken off the market, diabetics can still prepare such items at home, using saccharine along with natural and artificial flavors. Saccharine itself will remain available even if its use in commercial food preparations is discontinued.

Since it is important for adults who must care for, teach or otherwise deal with diabetic children to understand the problems that may arise—the possible dangers—and to have other valid information, both the American Diabetes Association and the Juvenile Diabetes Foundation have prepared specially printed material which the child can give to the teacher, scout leader, camp counselor, and so on. The same organizations have provided meeting-places where diabetic young people can gather and have "rap sessions" about their problems and how they solved them, and conduct other activities. These groups can be particularly useful to adolescents.

There is one particular misconception which can create

a vast number of problems by adding to the existing restrictions on the child's life. This is the belief that children with diabetes are more susceptible to infection than others.

This is not true. The juvenile or young adult diabetic who takes insulin is no more prone to infection than anyone else. Cuts, wounds, bruises, and fractures heal just as rapidly and as well as with non-diabetics. It is only with the approach of late middle age that the balance changes.

Parents often wonder whether or not they should send the child to a diabetic camp for the summer holiday.

The answer to this depends upon the child and his adjustment to the disease. If the child has not adjusted to the diabetes, if he feels isolated or unique, if he seems overly dependent in handling his urine tests and other chores, then a diabetic camp might be very helpful.

It will bring him into contact with other diabetics and thus reduce his feeling of isolation. It will teach him to test his urine, take his insulin and generally make him better able to manage his disease.

For the child with a good attitude toward his disease, a diabetic camp is not advised. Instead he would be better off in a regular camp with his everyday friends where he would learn, as he must, to function in a non-diabetic world.

The diabetic child, even one whose treatment is relatively flexible and whose family adjustment is on the highest level, will show signs of resentment and rebellion as he grows older. He will discover that his urine tests do not immediately show a rise in sugar even if he takes a forbidden chocolate or eats a helping of ice cream on the sly. At other times, his sugar may rise even though he has had absolutely no extras.

All this will make him question the validity of the restrictions—and he will begin to violate them, striving as

far as possible to do the things other children are permitted to do. If the parent-child relationship is a good
one, this rebellion should not get out of hand and will
probably be amenable to adjustment. If the relationship
is a bad one or the treatment has been too rigid, the rebellion could persist with serious consequences.

A doctor of the old school, who believed in rigid control, treated a number of child diabetics at a noted Mid-
western clinic. Each week the children reported for examination and, as part of the practice, presented carefully kept charts showing the results of the urine tests
they gave themselves daily.

One of the patients, a pretty young lady of about 10,
showed remarkably good control, and her urine charts
were invariably excellent as far as sugar and acetone were
concerned. On the basis of general health and growth as
well as the showing of the urine tests, her progress was
so good that the doctor took understandable pride in the
excellence of his treatment.

One day the young lady appeared for examination.
When the doctor asked for her urine chart she started to
hand it over then abruptly pulled it back. "Oh, no," she
blurted, "that's next week's chart. Here's this week's."

The doctor was so shocked that his belief in his treatment was shattered. The girl had obviously broken his restrictive rules, had been eating foods forbidden to her and
had then falsified her test charts to cover up her rebellion.
Despite this, her physical condition seemed fine and she
was showing all of the appearances of good control. There
was nothing the doctor could do to restore his position—
either in his own eyes or in the girl's.

This anecdote is not intended to prove that the child
who rebels against restrictions and flagrantly violates a
regimen will be better off for it. On the contrary.

But it does show that urine tests are not always true,

that, even when true, they are not always an accurate reflection of the diabetes situation; and that a certain amount of dietary leeway is possible without irreparable damage being done.

Revolt against authority is part of the normal process of growing up. In the diabetic child, it has an additional spur. The intelligent parent must understand this, anticipate it and be prepared to compensate for it with additional insulin or whatever else might be indicated.

About the best that can be hoped for is to have the rebellion minimized and kept within bounds. This goal can best be attained where the family relationships are good and where the treatment is balanced between the needs of the ailment and the human needs of the child.

CHAPTER 12

The Diabetic Adolescent

Adolescence is a time of great change and upheaval. Diabetes acquired in this period is the juvenile form with its explosive onset and tendency toward ketosis.

Diabetic or not, the adolescent grows at a prodigious rate, and the total need for calories is greater than at any other time of life. Equally great is the expenditure of calories to fill the vast demand for energy.

Adolescence is also a time when the activity of the endocrine glands is at its peak. The dynamic changes begun at puberty rise to a crescendo and involve the pituitary, the thyroid, the adrenal, and other glands. This is probably responsible for the increased incidence of diabetes in this period.

Emotionally, the adolescent swings wildly between childhood and adulthood. There is great instability as the personality seeks to adjust itself. It is a period of touchiness and sensitivity, of resentment and rebellion against the controls imposed upon the child by the adult world. The adolescent is in constant battle to assert himself and to win the right to make his own decisions regarding his life—and the only way this is ultimately done is by casting off parental control.

The problems of adolescence produce great conflicts both within the adolescent himself and also with his environment. This is true for all youngsters who have stopped being children but are not yet adults. Not only do they break with the past, they must also find the future

—and this is almost always beset with questions, fears and uncertainties.

Often, the family's mishandling of the diabetic child's adjustment problem will exacerbate rebellion. Typical is the case of a 14-year-old boy who had already been arrested three times and was awaiting trial for a fourth offense. The well-meaning parents of this boy—attempting to follow the rigid rules laid down by the original physician—had separated the child from the rest of the family at mealtimes. His table was set up in the outside hall; the refrigerator was locked and he alone denied a key; he had no spending money allowance such as was given his younger siblings.

Once this was changed, and the patient allowed to join the family at mealtimes—and given spending money as well as free access to the refrigerator—this potentially tragic situation was corrected.

Today, almost 30 years later, this patient is a respected and successful businessman, married, and with a family of his own.

Physical Problems of Diabetic Adolescents

Difficult as all this is for the normal teen-ager, the diabetic adolescent has the additional problems imposed by his disease. In the face of these new complexities, the care of adolescent diabetes becomes much more difficult than childhood diabetes.

First of all, and this seems a frightening thing to most parents, there is a very steep rise in the need for insulin. Daily requirements of 80 to 100 units are common. Parents ought not be disturbed by this—it is perfectly normal within the diabetes framework. Later, as the adolescent becomes an adult, the need for insulin will usually decline.

It should not be hard to understand why adolescents need more insulin than children or adults. Two factors are involved—calories and hormones.

In adolescence, metabolic activity is greater than at any other time. Growth demands greater caloric intake. At seventeen, a boy needs about 4,000 calories daily, almost twice what he will need as an adult. Most of these calories are taken as carbohydrates—bread, potatoes, cereals and the like, as well as fruits, ice cream, cake, and puddings. This in itself brings a sharp rise in the need for insulin.

The adolescent will spill more sugar into the urine despite the increased insulin. This, too, is perfectly normal and, in view of the huge carbohydrate consumption, should not worry parents unduly, provided the adolescent is growing well and shows none of the other diabetes symptoms.

Hormones are the other major reasons for the adolescent's big insulin need. As endocrine activity rises with adolescence, more hormones are poured into the blood—pituitary growth hormone, thyroid hormone, and sex hormones. These substances tend to inhibit the activity of insulin and therefore more is needed to make up for the reduced efficiency.

Girls sometimes have an additional problem imposed by the endocrine changes that come with puberty. Regardless of the over-all rise in insulin need, menstruation may make an even further demand. The adolescent girl diabetic may find that starting about two days before the onset of her period she will need a larger dose of insulin. This increased dose will have to be maintained until about the second day of her period, then it can usually be brought back to normal. The rise and fall of insulin need in conjunction with the menstrual cycle may continue until the menopause.

Emotional Problems of Diabetic Adolescents

The impact of social and emotional problems upon diabetes is greater in adolescence than at any other time of life. And the diabetes, in its turn, has an equally disturbing effect upon the social and emotional adjustments of the adolescent.

The adolescent is more fervid about his rights and independence than the child or adult. Parental interference is particularly resented, since it is a symbol of childhood that the adolescent strives to shatter.

As he attempts to assert himself, the adolescent diabetic often uses his diabetes as a weapon of rebellion against his parents. He may run away from home without taking his insulin equipment with him. He may be slipshod about taking insulin. There may be a sudden resistance to the testing of urine.

The urine tests are a special problem to adolescent girls during menstruation. They frequently refuse to take any tests during the period. Here the understanding of the parents and the intelligent explanations of the physician are vital. Urine tests are essential in the treatment of adolescent diabetes and must not be discontinued for any reason.

Another form of adolescent resistance is that of going on an overnight date and delaying the morning insulin injection until the return home. With the disposable equipment now available and the stability of insulin at room temperature, this need not occur.

One girl of sixteen, who lived in a rather unfortunate home environment and felt rejected by her mother, used her diabetes as a means of escaping from home. Whenever the situation became unbearable, she would stop taking her insulin injections and go into severe ketosis. Her next stop would be the hospital where the care, attention, and treatment would restore her sense of personal value.

She liked the hospital so much that as soon as she was up and about, she would offer to help the nurses and do other things to make herself useful. After a number of these hospitalizations she became a nurses' aid and came to the hospital to live.

Parents should recognize that rebellion is a normal stage of adolescence whether or not diabetes is involved. They should not become panicked and try to over-control the adolescent or impose rigid restrictions. Usually this will only intensify the resistance. In most cases, the best way to deal with the situation is with tolerance and understanding. The adolescent should be allowed to express his individuality with an absolute minimum of interference. If the parent-child relationship has been a good one in the past, the chances are that the stage of adolescent rebellion will come and go with little, if any, disturbance to treatment.

Adolescent Patient Must Treat Himself

It is very important for parents to understand that full responsibility for all phases of diabetes control *must* rest with the adolescent patient. This is equally true whether the diabetes stems from childhood or is newly acquired. The parents must yield *completely* all of the daily chores relating to the disease.

Unless this is done, the revolt may either take a more serious turn or the adolescent may fail to mature properly. He may become overly dependent and unable to face the problems of adulthood.

Where the parent is mistrustful of the child's ability to handle the disease and tries to exercise control indirectly or secretly, the adolescent is bound to sense it and become infuriated.

A mother, fearful that her diabetic son might go into insulin shock without anyone close knowing what to do, told her son's closest friend that her boy was diabetic. Swearing the friend to secrecy, she asked him to look out for the signs of insulin reaction and give her son candy or sugar when they occurred.

The next time they were at a party, the diabetic seemed to act a little light-headed while he was dancing with a girl; and the friend rushed over with candy. The diabetic boy, even though he was in the initial stage of an insulin reaction, knew immediately that the friend had been told his secret. And he also knew that the one who betrayed him could only be the parent.

That marked the end of the friendship; and the diabetic, fearful of further betrayals from his parents, hid his friendships from them and became even more withdrawn and secretive.

Bad as this situation is with boys, it is infinitely worse where the diabetic is a girl. For the adolescent girl, intensely conscious of her competition with other girls for the attention of boys and possible husbands, diabetes seems a tremendous handicap which must be kept secret. For a parent to divulge this secret to a close friend—who can only be a close competitor as well—would be unforgivable.

Parents must realize that secrecy is important to many adolescent diabetics during a stage of their growing up. The most intelligent thing they can do, with the assistance of the physician, is to teach the adolescent the importance of letting someone in the circle of friends know about the diabetes.

The choice of who is to be told must be left to the

diabetic, and the parents should respect this right. Many emotional and social problems are involved in this choice. The adolescent girl, for instance, might feel far more secure if a close friend did *not* know about her diabetes. Instead she might choose to confide in one she does not view as a near competitor.

Frequently, adolescents who acquire diabetes are far better able to cope with the situation than their parents.

One such case occurred recently when a seventeen-year-old girl appeared at a doctor's office. Accompanying her were her mother and a procession of aunts. The fact that the girl had diabetes had already been determined.

While the doctor was examining the girl as a means of working out a pattern of treatment, the mother had an emotional outburst.

"Why couldn't this happen to me instead of my daughter?" she demanded tragically.

Despite herself the girl winced. The other relatives, in whispers just loud enough for the girl to overhear, asked such questions as: What will happen to her? How long will she live? Will she be able to marry? Will she be able to have children?

Fortunately, the girl had been going to boarding school. The doctor therefore advised that the girl return to school and take up her regular life with the addition of the insulin, the tests, and other necessities of treatment.

The girl did just that and handled herself extremely well. Later she reported that while she was at school her diabetes was no problem at all. It was only during vacations and holidays, when she returned to the emotionally charged home environment, that she was made self-conscious about her ailment.

Another problem of adolescent diabetes arises from the normal decline of communication between the growing child and the parent. The adolescent leaves the home, goes to school and spends increasingly more time away from home as he seeks to form a living pattern of his own.

Ordinarily this results in considerable anxiety on the part of any parent, but where the child is diabetic the situation may be much more serious. At this stage the parent should never attempt to *force* trust and communication. About the only fruit force can bear is hostility. On the other hand, if the parent's relationship with the child has been based on acceptance and understanding rather than on strict control and rigid obedience, the decline in parent-child communication may never become serious enough to create a major problem.

For the teen-ager, most of the childhood infections are no longer a danger. Colds and accidents, on the other hand, are problems but not necessarily serious ones. They result in a temporary increase in the need for insulin, which may differ with each individual. Diabetic boys also have a greater tendency toward acne, which may become a social problem.

Since adolescent girls become increasingly sedentary while boys become more active, the possibility of accident is more likely among boys. Despite the risk of injury and insulin shock, the diabetic adolescent should be encouraged to participate in sports and other physical activities. *Parents should not try to have diabetic children excused from gymnasium and athletic events.*

There are two important reasons for this. It is vital for the adolescent's morale and sense of social status to be allowed to engage in normal activities. Secondly, physical activity makes the insulin he takes more efficient.

All the adolescent must remember, to avoid the possibility of shock, is to eat a bar of chocolate or drink a coke before the game.

Diabetic children should be allowed to run, jump, play baseball, football, basketball, or hockey. It would be well for parents to note that in the grueling game of tennis, two of America's outstanding stars have been diabetic since childhood. They are Billy Talbert and Ham Richardson.

Along with sports, all other normal social activities should be encouraged. There is no reason why diabetic adolescents should be less able than non-diabetics to stay out late, stay with a friend overnight, or even take a weekend or a vacation away from home.

Altogether, in sports, social and other activities, diabetes should not be allowed to become a problem.

A new problem has arisen for teen-age diabetics because of the current drug situation. Many adolescent diabetics now fear to take trips out of the country because examination of their luggage may reveal hypodermic equipment, causing embarrassment and requiring explanations. For this reason, every diabetic should at all times carry an identification card that indicates his legal right to carry the syringes and needles.

Some young diabetics have been compelled by threats of force to turn over their equipment to drug addicts. This has been particularly true in some high schools. It should be emphasized that remarkably few diabetic youngsters are themselves drug addicts.

Questions That Disturb Diabetic Adolescents

As the diabetic adolescent grows older and faces approaching adulthood, new problems rise up to disturb him.

What kind of future will he have? Will he be able to marry? Will he be able to meet the responsibilities of adult life? What sort of profession or career could he look forward to? Will he have any problem completing his education? Will he find a satisfactory place in society?

Such problems are faced by all adolescents, diabetic or not. But there is a difference. For the diabetic the problems are intensified as he uses them, consciously or unconsciously, to dramatize himself and his situation.

Diabetic girls are specially prone to fear the future and anticipate all sorts of hardships and obstacles in the way of a normal life.

These fears are usually groundless or vastly exaggerated.

Diabetes *does not* interfere with a girl's normal physical development. Nor does it interfere with the menstrual cycle. Diabetes *will not* prevent her from fulfilling the responsibilities of marriage; it *will not* rule out motherhood.

The future awaiting the diabetic is generally no different from that of the non-diabetic. It depends upon the individual and his relationship to the world around him. Only in some jobs, which we will discuss shortly, will the diabetes make any difference at all.

Regardless of reassurances, a number of adolescents are bound by personality to be uncertain and insecure in face of the future. If they happen to be diabetic, the underlying insecurity is heightened.

This is generally reflected in relations with members of the opposite sex and is usually more frequent and intense among girls. Where the diabetic is fearful about being unequal, he will be timid and hesitant about dating and "going out." Certainly, he will be reluctant to let his date know about his diabetes.

"To tell or not to tell" is one of the thorniest problems affecting the adolescent diabetic.

No major issues are involved on a casual date and there

is no need to divulge one's diabetes. But if the dating is more serious and may turn into courtship, then the problem looms increasingly large. Ultimately, the diabetes must be revealed. The question is: When?

The diabetic with a wholesome attitude toward the disease and with no feeling of inferiority will probably tell about it at the start of courtship.

Those who are less secure will wait—and be torn by a sense of guilt for not telling. Girls often do not tell until the engagement is an accomplished fact.

Advice is neither possible nor practical. Each diabetic will do what his or her personality permits and can live with. The insecure diabetic will tell when the guilt over-balances the insecurity. The secure diabetic will tell as soon as it seems important.

There is one point about this that can validly be made. Where a courtship or engagement breaks up over diabetes, the overwhelming probability is that the relationship did not have a sound basis to start with. Where there is a good relationship, diabetes is not used as a *reason* for breaking it up. It is only used as an *excuse* to end an unsound relationship which probably would have broken up on some other pretext if the diabetes did not exist.

Diabetes is *not* a barrier to marriage. The percentage of marriages among diabetics is about the same as among non-diabetics. Some diabetics marry with ease; some have disappointing episodes, with the diabetes used as an excuse. But, eventually, they marry.

Parents of non-diabetics will often oppose the marriage of their child to a diabetic for "medical reasons." Not only are these "reasons" usually invalid, but where there is a genuine emotional attachment, this opposition will be unsuccessful. Where marriage is concerned, some parents may oppose the free choice of their children in any case and will seize upon the most obvious excuse to make their opposition seem valid.

With modern-day management of diabetes, there is every reason for the diabetic boy or girl to approach the possibility of marriage secure in the knowledge that he or she will be every bit as good a partner as the non-diabetic, physically, emotionally, socially, financially, and intellectually.

What Careers for the Diabetic?

As far as higher education is concerned, diabetes is no problem. It does not impair the intelligence and has no effect on the ability to learn. Many states have programs for diabetics who graduate from high school. Tuition may be provided to any college, graduate school, or technical school under this program. The applicant makes his own selection and if accepted under the program, submits the bill for tuition to the local branch of the State Division of Vocational Rehabilitation.

There is no restriction upon diabetics in college or professional schools. They may become nurses, doctors, lawyers, engineers or nuclear physicists, business administrators or bookkeepers for that matter.

Military service *is* closed to diabetics. In the event of conscription the diabetic boy *will not* be drafted into the armed forces and can therefore plan his education or career *without* worrying about the loss of several years.

While practically all of the professions and most jobs will be open to him, the young diabetic planning his future should recognize that certain fields remain blocked. A number of civil-service jobs, teaching for instance, are sometimes closed to diabetics. So are police, fire-department, and other hazardous jobs. He should, however, avoid accepting any job which might cause a hazard to him or to the public as a result of possible insulin reaction.

Diabetics who require insulin usually will not be able to get jobs operating public conveyances such as taxis, buses, trains and the like. They will be unable to become locomotive engineers, pilots of commercial aircraft or ship's officers. The reason is the possibility of insulin shock which, at a critical moment, might endanger the passengers.

The young diabetic should not be surprised if certain companies refuse him a job for no apparent reason *although they may claim that diabetes is not a factor.*

Actually, a number of outworn and threadbare prejudices still cling to some big-company employment practices. These are carry-overs from the old days when diabetics survived on semi-starvation diets and were consequently weak and not fully productive.

The prejudices are gradually disappearing and are bound to vanish completely when companies learn that with modern treatment the diabetic who eats well is as productive as the non-diabetic. As for the belief that diabetics are harder hit by infections and more prone to prolonged absenteeism—the advent of antibiotics has made infections such as pneumonia no more hazardous to diabetics than to non-diabetics. With modern drugs, intelligent care and long-acting insulin, the diabetic is as good a job risk as anyone else.

There is a further factor which may make some companies reluctant to employ diabetics. This is the matter of pensions. A number of civil-service and other organizations which have pensions or employees' insurance plans feel that diabetics may retire earlier than non-diabetics and thus make a smaller contribution to the pension or insurance fund.

Apart from these restrictions—which are not as extensive as they appear and many of which are being eased —the young diabetic can look forward to entering practically any profession for which he is qualified or taking virtually any position in business or industry.

His diabetes will have no appreciable effect upon his ability to compete with other young men or women for an education and a career.

Nor should it have any effect upon the diabetic's ability to achieve a successful marriage, win a respected place in society, and create a fruitful and attractive future.

CHAPTER 13

The Diabetic Adult

One of the many mysteries of diabetes is the way in which it varies with the age at which it is acquired. Not only does susceptibility increase as we get older, but the type of diabetes is usually milder.

This does not necessarily mean that the nature of the diabetes changes as the patient ages. The child with severe juvenile diabetes will have juvenile diabetes for the rest of his life. But the diabetes acquired at thirty is generally less severe than the diabetes acquired at ten. Furthermore, the problems of the disease change as the diabetic proceeds through the unfolding stages of his life.

One important fact about diabetes that *does not* change must be emphasized. At no point in the diabetic's life, from childhood to old age, should properly managed diabetes be considered a bar to the treatment of any illness or injury by medication, radiation, or surgery.

Many people fear that the treatment of other ailments may aggravate existing diabetes or that diabetes may impede the treatment of the ailment. *This is not true.* Where the diabetes is properly cared for, the diabetic can undergo any operation or take any medication as well as the non-diabetic. Allergy pills, cold tablets, vitamins, aspirin, and so on may be taken without concern.

However, cortisone and its derivatives and certain diuretics may affect diabetes. But, even here, if a diabetic needs these drugs for the treatment of arthritis, asthma, or some skin ailment, he may take them without danger, provided their possible ill effects are canceled by an increase in the insulin dose.

Since adulthood embraces that vast segment of life spanning from adolescence through old age, the problems of diabetes undergo significant changes along the way. The young adult, aged twenty to forty, has problems which differ markedly from those of the middle-aged adult of forty to sixty. And the problems of the middle-aged adult are hardly the same as those of the elderly, aged sixty and up. For this reason, each of the three major stages of adult life must be considered alone in terms of its own special character.

THE YOUNG ADULT

Diabetes is almost three times more frequent among young adults than among youngsters and represents a sort of transitional stage between the severe diabetes of the young and the mild diabetes of later adulthood. The acute onset typical of childhood is not as common. Ketosis and insulin shock are less frequent. The disease is generally more stable, less difficult to manage and less dependent on insulin.

About one-third of the cases of diabetes among young adults are acute, showing all of the classical symptoms of juvenile diabetes. Usually, these are recognized easily and quickly.

Another third of the cases also show the classical symptoms, but these are not as extreme or as disturbing.

The remaining third of the cases do not have the obvious symptoms, are not readily recognized and are generally detected casually during a physical examination for insurance, employment, or army induction. Among women, diabetes may be detected during pregnancy, which requires regular analysis of the urine.

Oddly, and here is another interesting facet of diabetes, those cases which show the classical symptoms will usually require insulin for treatment. This represents about two-thirds of young adult diabetics.

The remaining third—those cases which were more difficult to detect—can usually be managed with oral therapy or, if the patient is overweight, a return to and maintenance of normal weight.

Among obese young adults, a weight reduction which is maintained may sometimes seem tantamount to a cure. This should never be taken for granted because, as they get older, their supply of available natural insulin may be further reduced by stress and the aging process. Should this happen, the diabetes would flare up again.

Treatment for the young adult who requires insulin resembles that of the juvenile except that the doses are smaller, and a single injection is usually enough for the whole day. Only a small number of young adults require an extra dose of quick-acting insulin.

There are two reasons why the young adult needs less insulin than the adolescent. Since he has stopped growing, his caloric needs are less. Furthermore, his living pattern is more regular.

Even if he has an acute onset of the disease, the young adult need not necessarily be hospitalized but can often be treated without undue interruption of his normal routine. The proper dose of insulin can be worked out by the physician as he evaluates the patient's daily response.

While the frequency of shock and coma is reduced in young adults, they do occur and must be treated in the usual way.

Oversleeping is one of the frequent causes of insulin

reaction among young adults. After a hard week's work, those extra hours of sleep on Saturday or Sunday morning may look especially attractive. But should this cause a delay in breakfast, shock may result. The same is true of social drinking, an extra hole of golf, or anything else that might make him delay or miss a meal.

Unusual physical activity remains a danger. The normally sedentary man who digs up the garden on the weekend runs the risk of shock.

On the other hand, the man who does hard physical labor during the week and rests up over the weekend may run the risk of ketosis unless he increases his weekend insulin dose.

Where the young adult does not take insulin, but manages with either diet or oral drugs, the possibility of shock or coma is reduced. This enables him to face changes in social life, physical activity, and general routine without any great difficulty.

Apart from these relatively minor physical problems, the diabetes presents no great threat. The social and emotional problems which loom so large to the adolescent are almost non-existent for the young adult. Only in three areas do diabetic young adults face what appear to be serious problems—insurability, employability, and parenthood.

Of these, the matter of parenthood is by far the more upsetting.

Should Diabetics Have Children?

The question "Should diabetics have children?" actually consists of three subsidiary questions. These are: Can a diabetic have children? Can parenthood be dangerous to the diabetic? Will the diabetic parent have diabetic children?

The first two questions are easily answered. Today's adult diabetics, as a result of modern treatment of the disease, are normally fertile and *can* have children.

Parenthood poses no risk to either parent where one or both are diabetic. There is no threat to life, no aggravation of the disease. Diabetes in the husband in no way affects the pregnancy of the wife. Diabetes in the wife requires a closer attention and more careful supervision during the pregnancy. Beyond that it should cause no appreciable disturbance either to the woman or the childbearing.

The third question—whether diabetic parents will produce diabetic children—is more complex and requires a closer look at some widely accepted beliefs.

Heredity *does* play a part in the susceptibility to diabetes. Where a parent is diabetic, there is a greater chance of a diabetes-prone child being produced.

Where both parents are diabetic, there is a considerable risk of producing a diabetic child. But even this risk, while sizable, may not be as great as statistical prediction would indicate.

Genetically, the predisposition to diabetes is not as simple as once believed. More than 30 different genetic abnormalities, many of which are passed along as simple Mendelian traits, can produce disturbances in carbohydrate tolerance. Different genetic abnormalities have been found in juvenile-onset diabetes and maturity-onset diabetes, and the genetic patterns found in the young patients with maturity-onset diabetes—called MODYs by Fajans—differ from those in the JODYs—juvenile-onset diabetes in the young. To complicate the genetic picture still further, Dr. D. A. Pyke has found that in a sizable group of identical twins with diabetes, the age at onset often differed within twin pairs.

Since there are so many modes of possible inheritance,

Drs. D. L. Remoin and J. Zonana, who are conducting genetic studies at U.C.L.A., warn that it would be incorrect to counsel diabetic patients on the basis of one mode. For this reason alone, accurate genetic counseling is not presently possible for the majority of patients. About all that can be said safely is that diabetes occurs more frequently in families with an appreciable history of diabetes.

In view of all this, should diabetics have children?

Yes, where one of the parents is diabetic.

Where both parents are diabetic, there should be considerably more weighing of the pros and cons. But even in those cases it is impossible to be dogmatic. People who want children enough and can have them, often will have them regardless of statistical risks.

Insurance for the Diabetic

Apart from the problems of parenthood—and employability, which was discussed in the chapter on the adolescent diabetic—the young adult faces the intensely practical problem of insurability. This could be of considerable moment where the diabetic is concerned with protecting his family against accident, illness, or death.

Today's diabetic need have no great worry about insurance. Until the mid-1940s, insurance companies rejected all diabetic applicants for life insurance. This rejection was based in great part on the prejudices and attitudes that had developed in the pre-insulin era. In more recent years, dozens of companies have taken another look at diabetes in terms of modern treatment. As a result there has been a complete change in attitude.

The diabetic who wants life insurance today can obtain it from a number of companies. But, as with anyone suffering a chronic ailment, his premium will be higher.

Diabetics can also have accident, health, hospitalization, and disability insurance at no increased premium, *but only as members of a group insurance plan*. Individual insurance of this type will be extremely difficult, if not impossible, for diabetics to obtain at present.

Many diabetics may also find it useful to know that the Veterans Administration has recognized diabetes acquired during military service as justification for a disability pension. This pension can be obtained even where the diabetes develops *after* the discharge from service— *but no later than within one year afterward.*

It should also be noted that in most states, diabetics who apply for a driver's license must present a letter from their physician stating that the public would not be endangered if the diabetic were permitted to drive. The physician's judgment is based on the patient's susceptibility to insulin reaction. Where reaction is relatively rare and quickly checked, the diabetic driver should present no risk.

Beyond the impact of these major factors of parenthood, employability and insurability, the non-medical problems of diabetes are probably less for the young adult than for anyone else. Diabetes seems less threatening to him than to the adolescent who fears what will happen when he has to face the world on his own; or to the middle-aged or elderly diabetic over whom the fear of death casts a lengthening shadow.

For the young adult, the fulfillment of work, a career, and the raising of a family provide positive goals and incentives possessed by none of the other groups. He is more concerned with problems of achievement than of ailment.

One further point should be made regarding employability. If a diabetic can no longer pursue the same line of work as before because of his disease, he can apply to the Division of Vocational Rehabilitation for help in retraining for a new job or career. Under a Federal program of grants in aid to the chronically ill, each state is charged by law with responsibility for providing such aid without cost to eligible applicants.

THE MIDDLE-AGED DIABETIC

Between the ages of forty and sixty, diabetes becomes vastly more frequent and considerably less severe than in earlier years.

In middle age, the incidence of diabetes is almost ten times greater than among young adults. It also becomes about twice as frequent among women as men.

The number of middle-aged diabetics who show the obvious symptoms of the disease amounts to about half of the cases—considerably less than among young adults where two out of three have the classical symptoms.

These are the acute cases, and practically all once required insulin injections. Today, only about 50 percent still need insulin; the rest can do well on oral drugs.

The remaining diabetics, half of the middle-aged total, do not have the obvious symptoms and the disease is usually detected during an examination for something else. In this group, if the patient is obese, a weight-reduction and maintenance diet is usually sufficient to control the disease. Where the patient is not obese, insulin or oral drugs may be needed.

Of all middle-aged diabetics, about 50 percent require insulin for treatment. The remaining 50 percent can be managed with diet or oral therapy alone.

Since the need for insulin is usually a direct indication of the severity of diabetes, the middle-age type is patently less severe than the younger forms. There is less ketosis, less coma, and fewer incidents of shock. But stress, illness, accident, or surgery may increase the severity of the ailment and cause a need for insulin where no such need existed before. Once the emergency is over, treatment can usually return to normal.

It is at this stage in life that the symptoms of aging begin to make themselves evident. The most common of these is arteriosclerosis—hardening of the arteries—which develops in the normal as well as in the diabetic population. Other ailments related to age also appear—coronary artery disease, hypertension, and strokes.

These ailments arise as part of the process of growing old. They are not unique to diabetics. But, where diabetes exists, they tend to occur somewhat sooner. It is as though diabetes accelerates the aging of the circulatory system. For this reason weight control is of particular importance to the middle-aged diabetic. Overweight— even mild overweight—seems to be a serious contributory factor in diabetes as well as in circulatory ills. A U.S. Public Health Service study shows that overweight individuals, whether or not they have a family history of diabetes, are more than twice as likely to become diabetic as people of normal weight.

Since all this is a problem affecting the total population at this age, there is no special solution for the diabetic. A tremendous amount of research into the causes and possible prevention or cure of this group of ailments is currently being done. Sooner or later the answers will begin to take shape, and these will apply equally to the diabetics and the non-diabetics who cross the threshold into the middle years.

THE ELDERLY DIABETIC

Past the age of sixty there is a continued increase in the incidence of diabetes. It is three times as frequent as in middle age.

To balance this climb, there is a decline in the severity

of the disease. It is relatively mild in regard to urinary sugar, fewer cases require insulin, more can be managed with dietary control or oral drugs. There is also less ketosis and fewer incidents of insulin shock.

The disease itself seems to pose fewer difficulties, but the aging process creates a new set of problems in relation to the disease. So, while the possibility of shock is more remote, the consequences may be far more severe. Arteries become more brittle with age, and shock may now cause serious organic damage as a result—a heart attack or a stroke.

The elderly person, diabetic or not, is more prone to accident than in his middle years; more susceptible to certain illnesses; more likely to require surgery.

Where diabetes does exist, it should not be a problem interfering with proper treatment. But the stress of the acute illness, the accident or the operation may cause a change in the diabetes necessitating an increase of insulin or some other compensation in treatment.

For the elderly diabetic, the complications arising from arteriosclerosis are also more frequent and more severe than for the non-diabetic. Injury and infection, which caused no special problems for the younger diabetic, now are hazardous because of the decrease in blood circulation. Especially vulnerable are the feet, where circulation is usually most sluggish.

Special Precautions for Elderly Diabetics

There are a number of things the diabetic can do to protect himself from these complications of aging.

First of all, he can help his circulatory system by keeping his weight at normal or slightly below. Probably the best weight at this age is 10 percent below what is considered normal.

Equally important, he must take the proper precautions

to avoid injury and infection, especially of the feet. Here, the diabetic should exercise common sense and observe such injury-preventing rules as the following: He should avoid ill-fitting shoes. He should avoid socks that are too large, too small or wrinkled. They may cause blisters or other damage. He should not walk barefoot, thus avoiding splinters or other injuries. He should exercise extreme care cutting his toenails. He should not apply powerful antiseptics such as iodine to delicate tissues. He should not attempt to trim his own corns or bunions or use corn or bunion removers which may be caustic. He should avoid extremes of heat or cold. Hot footbaths or hot-water bottles, if too hot, can be as dangerous as frostbite. He should be especially aware of the importance of cleanliness and hygiene. Feet should be washed carefully, at least once each day. Socks should be changed at least as frequently. He should be careful in choosing his work or recreation, avoiding activities which may cause injury, especially to the feet. An upholsterer, who frequently stepped on tacks, suffered serious complications. So did a night watchman on a building project after his feet became soaked in mud, then chilled. Equally hazardous are tasks involving the movement of heavy objects which may strike the feet.

These are some of the more obvious precautions. They should suggest others, fitted to each diabetic's individual pattern of living. Most important of all, the elderly diabetic should never attempt to treat injury or infection on his own. This should be left strictly to the physician.

Close contact with the doctor is vital at every stage of diabetes and is particularly important for the elderly patient. In any situation of stress, injury, infection, or even where the slightest doubt or worry arises, the physician should be contacted at once.

The emotional problems of the elderly diabetic are in

no way different from those of the non-diabetic. They usually center about a growing feeling of isolation and loneliness, a greater concern with death. There are no capsule solutions for these problems, depending as they do upon individual needs in relation to individual environments.

Any activity or situation which involves the elderly person and gives him a sense of continuing purpose is usually helpful. Anything which tends to further his isolation or a sense of declining usefulness is harmful.

The woman who tells her aging mother that she need no longer strain her eyes knitting sweaters for the grand children may unwittingly be causing great harm by destroying her mother's sense of being needed.

Old or young, diabetics have the same problems as other people their age in addition to the problems which may be unique to the disease. Except where the diabetes creates distinctly special needs, they should be treated like any other human being. In this way the diabetic will be free to live, love, work and function to the fullest capacity possible.

CHAPTER 14

Diabetes as a Special Problem for Women

Although diabetes spares neither of the sexes, it poses some special problems for the female.

For one thing, diabetes seems to have a particular affinity for women. Of the estimated 4,500,000 diabetics in the United States, more than 2,500,000 are female. What is more, of every 100 women and girls alive today, more than four are due to become diabetic.

The precise reasons for this are not fully known, although it seems virtually certain that metabolic and endocrine factors relating to childbearing and menopause are involved. Mothers, as has already been shown, are more susceptible than non-mothers; and, after the age of forty-five, women become twice as susceptible as men.

The fact that diabetes prefers women is not the only characteristic making it a special problem for the wife and mother. Women must take greater care in managing the disease than men. This is true for physiological reasons as well as for reasons arising from the everyday demands imposed upon the woman who must make a home and raise a family.

Finally, there is that most uniquely feminine complication of all to add to the problems of diabetes—that of pregnancy.

Before the advent of insulin and modern treatment, fertility was extremely low and diabetic women were rarely able to achieve pregnancy. Today the situation is completely reversed. With proper treatment, the diabetic woman is as fertile as the normal woman and has an equally high probability of surviving the pregnancy. What is more, where the chances of successful pregnancy were about nil in the pre-insulin era, today they have risen to better than 80 percent and, as treatment improves, will go even higher.

Non-diabetic women suffer a 4 percent loss of infants between the sixth month of pregnancy and the second day after birth. With diabetic mothers, where treatment is on a high level, the loss is only 6 percent higher.

The problems of pregnancy as they affect the diabetes are not particularly complex but they do demand careful attention.

Regardless of previous treatment, during pregnancy the diabetic will require both diet and insulin and the control must be much more meticulous than usual.

Morning sickness, which is common during the first three months of pregnancy, may carry a threat of acidosis or insulin reaction. While serious to the mother, this can be far more dangerous to the unborn child. As a measure of protection, the prospective mother must be sure to take adequate nourishment. Where she has any difficulty with food or anything else, she must notify her physician at once.

In light of the newer knowledge that high blood sugar reduces the oxygen-carrying capacity of the hemoglobin, something which may have an adverse effect on the fetus, it is more important than ever to maintain blood sugar levels as close to normal as possible. This may require several insulin injections daily. Pregnancy often sends the insulin requirements into unpredictable gyrations; the needed amount may rise to as much as two or three times that usually taken in about two-thirds of the women, and remain stationary or drop in the other third. For these reasons regular urine and blood tests for sugar and acetone become extremely important.

Ordinarily, we expect that insulin requirements will continue to mount with each succeeding month of pregnancy until the time of delivery. A drop in insulin need, therefore, is regarded as a possible sign of fetal distress.

The pregnant diabetic has a greater tendency to spill sugar into the urine. This is not as significant as in the non-pregnant diabetic, but should be watched. Far more important would be the presence of acetone, which must be corrected without delay.

The diabetic woman has a greater-than-normal tendency to retain water in her tissues during pregnancy. For this reason a low-salt diet is usually important.

Where the diabetes has been well-treated, childbirth is more nearly normal. Stress, family and economic background are important factors. The woman with a good home environment usually has an easier time. The woman whose diabetes is relatively recent has a better chance of successful pregnancy than the woman with diabetes of twenty years or more.

Until about ten years ago, there was a much higher rate of infant loss among diabetics before, during and soon after birth. There was a higher percentage of spontaneous abortions and miscarriages. A number of infants seemed to develop well until about four weeks *before* birth, then they died in the womb for reasons still unknown. Another difficulty arose from the fact that diabetes in the mother often made the child too large for an easy or successful delivery.

Today, as the result of careful teamwork on the part of the mother's physician who cares for the diabetes, the obstetrician who attends to the pregnancy and delivery, and the pediatrician who cares for the infant after birth, there has been a dramatic improvement in the number of successful pregnancies.

New Approaches Help Successful Pregnancy

One of the most important contributions is made by a somewhat different approach to delivery. Instead of waiting for the pregnancy to run its full course, the baby is delivered before it either grows too large or dies in the womb during the last weeks of gestation.

The best time for delivery is usually during the 36th or 37th week of pregnancy, about 3 to 4 weeks before the normal time of birth. The optimum moment, which would allow for the fullest development of the infant as well as the best chance for a successful delivery, is determined by the obstetrician, usually in consultation with the mother's physician.

A number of new techniques are now available to help determine the best time for delivery. One of these is the use of sonography—high-frequency sound waves—in place of X-ray. Since the ultrasound has none of the hazards of X-ray and provides a somewhat similar picture with which the size and position of the fetus and placenta can be monitored, it can be performed as often as needed.

A second new guide to the proper moment for delivery

is provided by measurement of the hormone estriol, which is secreted into the mother's blood in increasing amounts as the pregnancy progresses. This hormone can now be measured in both blood and urine, and, should a sudden drop in estriol secretion be noted, the infant is delivered as soon as possible.

In addition to these procedures, there is now a method of determining the development of the fetus' ability to breathe on its own should the baby be delivered. By a technique known as amniocentesis, the doctor removes a sample of amniotic fluid from the mother's uterus and tests it for its content of lecithin and sphyngomyelin, two chemicals that reflect the state of development of the fetus' lungs. If the ratio of lecithin is high enough, the baby will be able to breathe; if it is too low, delivery should be delayed, since normal respiration will be less likely.

By these means, the fetus is allowed the fullest possible development, and the incidence of high-risk premature delivery has been reduced.

When the optimum moment for delivery is determined, normal labor may be induced by certain drugs or other methods, or the baby may be delivered by Caesarean section. However it is accomplished, the technique of planned delivery has made it possible for the vast majority of diabetic women to achieve successful pregnancies. Then, with the pediatrician standing by to take over at birth, even the borderline infant has a good chance of survival.

At Mount Sinai Hospital in New York, during a 25-year period ending in 1976, more than 4,000 pregnant diabetics were cared for. Receiving the best of modern "team" treatment involving the physician, obstetrician, and pediatrician, they produced a better than 94 percent record of successful births.

Although the improvement has been enormous, successful pregnancy still remains a greater challenge for the diabetic than for the non-diabetic woman. Among the things making motherhood more difficult for the diabetic is the tendency toward earlier atherosclerosis and an accelerated aging of certain organs. Thus, a diabetic woman in her twenties seems to have the same problems as a non-diabetic woman in her forties. The overall loss of infants from all causes during pregnancy and shortly after birth is about the same in both groups.

We have indeed come a long way from the pre-insulin era, when pregnancy for the diabetic was most often either impossible or fatal.

Other Special Problems of Diabetic Women

Pregnancy is only one of the physiological problems that may complicate the diabetes of women.

Some diabetic women may have premenstrual difficulty. If they require insulin there may be a rapid rise in the needed dose shortly before menstruation; a sharp drop during or immediately after the period.

The menopause, with all its dynamic stresses, causes further changes and problems. At this time of life the tendency toward obesity seems to increase in women to a greater degree than in men. Since overweight can seriously complicate the diabetes, it becomes more important for women to watch their calories.

From young adulthood on, fungus infections in the genital area are more common among women. These can cause serious itching and discomfort. Where they exist, they can be treated with special fungicides which the physician will prescribe. Special hygienic care can also help prevent them.

As the diabetic woman enters middle age she becomes more susceptible than the man to bladder, kidney, and other urinary infections. Once these were a serious problem. Today, with a wide range of antibiotics at the disposal of the physician, the infections are amenable to control.

Diabetes also seems to increase a woman's vulnerability to heart ailments. Ordinarily, the healthy woman is three times *less* likely than a man to suffer from heart disease. Diabetes wipes out this advantage and makes the woman equally assailable.

Considering all these physiological factors, it is quite clear that even if everything else were equal, diabetes poses a greater problem for women than men.

Everything else is *not* equal if the woman is also a wife, and even less equal if she is a mother.

The average man lives a fairly regular life. He rises at a given time, eats at given times, has about the same amount of activity each day at his job. The very fact of a regular job usually imposes a set of regular habits which can be very helpful in the control of diabetes.

The wife, especially if she is also a mother, has an irregular life. Household emergencies are always arising to complicate the management of her disease.

A child takes sick and has to be treated at once.

Perhaps the child is hurt at outdoor play, and the mother has to fetch him home just as she is starting a required meal.

Her husband calls up about a last-minute dinner guest, so she has to run out for some emergency shopping.

These and events like them occur almost daily to upset the regularity of a housewife's life.

If she is taking insulin and these irregularities make her delay a meal or engage in too much physical activity, she may suffer a reaction. Even the best-organized homemaker cannot anticipate and be ready for all emergencies of cleaning, cooking, shopping, and child-raising.

Where the diabetic is a young adult, these problems are much more significant. Not only is it more likely that she will require insulin, but she is also more likely to be in the flush of building a family—a situation fairly bristling with emergencies and potential hazards.

On the other hand, this is not the case where the diabetes is controlled by diet alone or where oral therapy can supplant the need for insulin injections. Under those conditions, the problems lose their significance, since the diabetic woman is enabled to function more flexibly in the changing situations of daily life.

Looking back over the full range of diabetes problems as they affect women, the changes wrought by insulin and the over-all improvement of treatment have opened a whole new world of possibilities.

Because of these advances, the woman with diabetes is almost every bit as able as her non-diabetic sister to meet the responsibilities, emergencies, and pleasures of being a wife, a mother, and everything else that womanhood implies.

PART FOUR

The Prospects

CHAPTER 15

On the Threshold of Tomorrow

Up until about a century ago mankind was afflicted by a widespread disease known as *The Fever*. This strange malady showed certain peculiar variations. Some victims passed it off with scarcely any disturbance in their daily living. Others died. Regardless of the variations, one symptom was always present—the rise in temperature that gave the disease its name.

Treatment of The Fever consisted of lowering the temperature to normal. This involved the use of drugs similar to aspirin, sweating, purging, bleeding, and other practices then in vogue. In a great many cases the treatment was successful and the patients recovered.

Today we know that there was no such disease as The Fever. It was a catch-all designation for a whole range of fever-producing infections all the way from a severe cold to malaria, meningitis, typhoid, and pneumonia. We also know that each of these ailments, although they all produce the common symptoms of fever, is caused by a different microbe. Each of these microbes, in turn, is treated with specific antibiotics or other agents; and, once the cause is removed, the fever and other disease symptoms will vanish.

Today's diabetes resembles The Fever of a century ago in many respects. It shows considerable variation, but in practically every case there is a common symptom—a tendency to abnormally high blood sugar. Treatment does not strike at the cause of the particular variety of diabetes involved. Instead it seeks to check the major symptom by reducing the sugar levels of the blood and urine.

Perhaps a century from now physicians will look back at us, shake their heads with benign tolerance and say:

"What the physicians of the mid-Twentieth century called diabetes was really a whole range of ailments, each with a different set of causes but with one symptom in common—abnormally high blood sugar. Since they couldn't distinguish between the causes of the different ailments, they could neither prevent nor cure them. Instead they treated the common symptom, using various means to keep the blood and urine sugar under control."

Considering how little we actually do know about the causes of diabetes, we have made remarkable progress in controlling the symptoms of the disease ever since the isolation of insulin. We have also developed a clearer understanding of some of the variations that make one case of diabetes differ from another.

Diabetes Research Revitalized

In the years between the introduction of insulin and the discovery of the oral drugs, there was a sluggishness in diabetes research as well as a rigidity in thinking about this disease. To many, the problem was as good as solved since the ailment in most cases could be fairly well controlled by insulin injections and diet. Consequently, interest in continued research and in the expansion of understanding waned.

During this period it was believed that every diabetic had an absolute deficiency of insulin.

Then, when the first sulfonylurea was introduced and showed that sulfonylurea drugs might be effective for a large number of adult diabetics, the prevailing lethargy was abruptly swept aside. A whole new group of investigators in all parts of the world turned their attention to the questions raised by the oral drugs.

It was obvious, for instance, that these drugs were not insulin and had no insulinlike activity. Yet, the response they produced in the patient was one that could only occur in the presence of active insulin. Therefore it seemed clear that many of these diabetic patients *did* have insulin. However, it was somehow deficient or inactivated in the disease state but could be stimulated into activity by the drug.

The Glucagon Role

Even this picture of diabetes, somewhat more sophisticated than the earlier concepts, turned out to be overly simplified and had to be altered drastically as new discoveries began to proliferate during the first half of the 1970s.

Instead of diabetes being due simply to a failure of insulin production or activity, it became clear that other hormones were equally involved in carbohydrate metabolism. Glucagon, which had been discovered in 1921, came under intensive study by Dr. R. H. Unger of Dallas.

What made this and a number of other advances possible was a monumental breakthrough in biomedical science—the development by S. A. Berson and R. S. Yalow of New York of the radioimmunoassay technique that made the detection and measurement of circulating insulin levels feasible. By this means they were able to show, among other things, abnormalities in insulin release and timing, and the presence of diabetes in patients whose pancreases were still producing insulin.

Using a modification of the Berson-Yalow technique, Dr. Unger and his colleagues were able to measure extremely small amounts of glucagon in blood and tissue. They found that in every diabetic, high sugar levels were always accompanied by rises in glucagon levels. And when sugar levels fell, so did glucagon. It seemed clear that glucagon, which was produced in the alpha cells of the pancreas as well as in the gastrointestinal tract, also had a role in the regulation of carbohydrate metabolism. Insulin was not the only factor.

However, some important questions remained to be answered. Did a rise in glucagon cause a rise in blood sugar? And if so, would control of glucagon have an effect on control of diabetes?

A means of answering these questions came in 1973 with the discovery, purification, and synthesis of another hormone, somatostatin, by R. Guillemin and his associates at the Salk Institute in La Jolla, California.

The following year, in Seattle, Dr. D. J. Koerker and her associates showed somatostatin to be a powerful suppressant of plasma glucagon. Infusing the newly-synthesized hormone into baboons, they observed a dramatic fall in glucagon levels.

These and other answers from researchers in a number of countries, backed by the results of his own investigations, led Dr. Unger to revive the theory of a single bihormonal regulator of carbohydrate metabolism, first proposed in 1907 by Dr. M. A. Lane. Dr. Unger suggested that the alpha and beta cells of the pancreas operate as a functional unit, with a balance between glucagon and insulin being maintained in normal situations.

In diabetics, both insulin-dependent and non-insulin dependent, abnormally high levels of glucagon were seen, particularly after a meal. These levels were difficult to restore to normal levels even with injections of insulin. In addition, high blood-sugar levels seemed to parallel the high glucagon levels. But when glucagon levels were reduced with somatostatin, blood sugar was also reduced and smaller doses of insulin were needed in those who were insulin-dependent.

As a result of these findings, Dr. Unger and a Swiss colleague, Dr. Lelio Orci, suggested that the hyperglycemia of diabetes was due not alone to the absolute or relative deficiency of insulin, as the traditional concept pictured. Instead, they proposed that insufficient insulin activity resulted in a decrease in glucose uptake by the cells. In addition, an elevated release of glucagon by the alpha cells stimulated the liver to release more glucose into the blood, resulting in hyperglycemia.

In support of this new concept of hyperglycemia, Drs. Unger and Orci pointed to three pieces of evidence. First of all, they noted that hyperglycemia did not occur naturally unless glucagon was present. Nor did hyperglycemia occur in animals that had been given enough somatostatin to suppress both insulin and glucagon. Finally, normal blood sugar levels could be achieved in human diabetics with a fixed dose of insulin if glucagon secretion had been suppressed by somatostatin.

Tests in this direction are continuing and expanding. If they fulfil their promise, somatostatin may help achieve a more precise control of diabetes than has been possible before. For the moment, however, it should be understood that somatostatin has only a brief period of activity, and, unless this could be prolonged, it would have to be administered almost continuously. Moreover, because it interferes with the action of growth hormone, it could not be used in children.

Recent research has also implicated other factors that

appear to be involved in producing diabetes, provided that the underlying genetic susceptibility is preesnt. One of these is the phenomenon known as autoimmunity, in which the body's disease-fighting mechanisms—the antibodies—turn against the body itself. In 1974, Dr. A. C. MacCuish and his associates in Edinburgh reported that they had detected antibodies to the pancreatic islets in five patients with insulin-dependent diabetes.

At Stanford University, in California, meanwhile, Dr. G. Reaven and his group have been working on a number of aspects of diabetes, including the question of autoimmunity. He has suggested that there appears to be a relationship between a certain group of inherited genes, HLA, and the appearance of insulin-dependent diabetes due to an autoimmune effect. Where a specific type of this gene is present, according to Dr. Reaven, certain kinds of virus may "cause a phenomenon whereby the body does not recognize itself and produces antibodies which destroy the insulin-producing beta cells of the pancreas."

This had been suggested by a British study by Drs. A. G. Cudworth and J. C. Woodrow of the University of Liverpool, which showed insulin-dependent diabetics to have a significantly increased incidence of HLA-A8 and HLA-W15 antigens than nondiabetic controls. Since the genes that determine immunologic responses and susceptibility to viral diseases are close to the HLA genes on the chromosome in certain animals, it is possible that these HLA types might predispose a person to diabetes by influencing virus receptors in the pancreas, or by adversely modifying the immunologic response to such viruses.

The Viral Link to Diabetes

The notion that a virus infection could be involved in the development of diabetes was first advanced in 1864 when Dr. J. Stang, a Norwegian physician, reported that diabetes appeared in one of his patients shortly after a mumps infection. Since then, information linking diabetes to viral infections has been accumulating from many sources. Today, the entire question of such a link is being investigated by several groups in the United States and abroad, and considerable evidence has been found to suggest that some viruses do indeed attack the beta cells and impair or destroy their insulin-secreting capability.

The evidence, as far as human diabetes is concerned, consists of a growing number of reports of diabetes following viral disease, as well as epidemiologic or population studies showing a relationship between "outbreaks" of diabetes in an area and recent viral infection. Strongly supporting this evidence are the results of a number of experimental animal studies.

The epidemiologic evidence has come from as widely scattered sites as Sri Lanka, Great Britain, and the Buffalo-Rochester area in New York.

In Sri Lanka (formerly Ceylon) 15 children were studied by Dr. J. E. J. Aiyathurai following infections of the upper respiratory tract with Coxsackie B virus. The children all had developed ketoacidosis, and tests were undertaken to determine the cause. The results indicated that in a number of the children the ketoacidosis was due to a diminished glucose tolerance, which, Dr. Aiyathurai suggested, resulted from a transient inhibition of the glucose carrier system.

In Great Britain, Drs. D. R. Gamble and K. W. Taylor, and their associates, studying patients with recently detected insulin-dependent diabetes, found that within a period of three months after the diagnosis there was a significantly higher level of antibodies to Coxsackie B virus than could be seen in nondiabetics or in patients with longstanding diabetes.

Further evidence was provided by the British Diabetes Association, which began a registry of all newly-diagnosed juvenile diabetics in December, 1972. Their data show the seasonal incidence of diabetes to be similar to that of the total incidence of childhood viral infections, with an autumn peak due to enteroviral infections and a winter peak due to respiratory infections.

The British scientists Gamble and Taylor, in addition to finding an epidemiologic link between Coxsackie B virus infection and the onset of diabetes, reported that the infection was followed by either partial and transient damage to the beta cells or total and permanent destruction. Some children recovered from the diabetes; some did not. It might be speculated from this that some of the remissions seen in children are really recoveries from partial viral damage to the beta cells. These cells would remain at risk, however, and could be more readily destroyed by some stress later in life.

In Buffalo, Dr. H. A. Sulz has reported a series of studies which showed that epidemics of mumps in New York's Erie County could be related to the development of juvenile-type diabetes several years later, with an average lag period of 3.8 years. This lag, he suggested, may reflect the time necessary for the mumps virus to produce permanent damage to the beta cells.

It is possible that pancreatic injury caused by many different viral infections are additive, and the clinical appearance of diabetes would be linked only to the most recent infection, although most of the damage might have been caused by a number of earlier infections.

Evidence from a wide range of sources, reported over a period of years, has linked the development of numerous cases of insulin-dependent diabetes to mumps, rubella (German measles), and other viral infections.

Experiments Support Epidemiologic Findings

Strong support for the virus-diabetes link comes from a number of animal studies in which pancreatic damage and diabetes have actually been produced by viral infections.

Probably the most extensive work in this area has been done with the encephalomyocarditis (EMC) virus in mice. Dr. J. E. Craighead and his group at the University of Vermont have shown that a strain of this virus can produce a disease in mice very similar to juvenile diabetes in humans. These observations have been confirmed in experiments by Drs. A. L. Notkins and D. W. Boucher at the National Institutes of Health, who also found a genetic tendency, controlled by more than one gene, to develop diabetes as a result of this viral infection.

Craighead has also shown that if mice genetically resistant to diabetes were given EMC virus and then cortisone or testosterone, they lost their resistance and their beta cells were destroyed. This might suggest that the peak periods of diabetes in humans—puberty, pregnacy, and menopause—are related to the significant hormonal changes acting in conjunction with some other etiologic stimulus, such as, for instance, a virus capable of attacking the pancreas.

Using another virus, the Coxsackie B_4, Dr. Notkins and

his associates, Drs. K. Hayashi and M. E. Ross, showed that in mice, this particular viral strain also damaged the pancreas, but only the acinar portion which produces digestive enzymes. The islets of Langerhans were spared.

The virus of Venezuelan Equine Encephalitis (VEE), which, unlike the EMC virus, also attacks humans, was tested in mice, hamsters, and rhesus monkeys by Dr. E. J. Rayfield and his associates at the U.S. Army Medical Research Institute of Infectious Diseases in Frederick, Maryland. They found that this virus caused a severe decrease in insulin release, without impairing glucose tolerance, for up to six months following virus inoculation.

Dr. Rayfield, now at the Mount Sinai Medical Center in New York, has suggested that this phenomenon may represent a virus-induced prediabetes which, at a later stage, progresses to frank diabetes mellitus. It is also possible that the VEE virus acts upon other hormone systems in addition to insulin, perhaps glucagon or somatostatin. Should that be the case, it might explain why the insulin defect has not produced symptoms in these animals.

The rhesus monkey studies may prove particularly fruitful since these animals resemble humans and the disease process can be followed in them for an extended period. Since VEE also affects humans, research is being planned by Dr. Rayfield, in collaboration with Dr. G. S. Bowen of the Public Health Service, to determine whether there may be a link between that viral infection and diabetes in humans.

The research in this area is gaining considerable momentum, and, should the viral hypothesis be confirmed, the next step would be the development of safe, killed-virus vaccines for those viral infections that may contribute to the onset of diabetes mellitus.

Insulin Resistance and Receptor Sites

Researchers are presently clarifying another apparent cause of non–insulin-dependent diabetes, one that was previously referred to as insulin resistance. Most of the maturity-onset diabetics, as we know, produce normal or even excessive amounts of insulin, yet this insulin, for some reason, encounters a reduced sensitivity at the target cells, where it is supposed to produce its effect. In short, it is there, but it does not work efficiently. While the precise cause is still to be discovered, some solid clues to the underlying defect have been revealed in the past few years.

It was discovered that there are certain sites on the membranes of cells to which specific hormones attach themselves to perform their biologic tasks. A good analogy here would be the lock and key, with the lock representing the receptor site and the hormone the key—and only a certain type of key being able to fit a particular lock.

Studies of insulin receptors began in 1949 when W. C. Stadie of the University of Pennsylvania attempted to determine the interaction between the hormone and its receptor by using radioactively tagged insulin. Because of a number of technical difficulties, success eluded him, but he had opened a path for further investigation.

By the mid 1970s, not only had insulin receptors been identified and carefully studied, but glucagon receptors had also been isolated. This work was performed by a number of distinguished scientists, among whom were I. J. Roth, J. M. Olevsky, and G. M. Reaven. A number of interesting findings were reported as a result of this world-wide investigation.

Roth, working as the National Institutes of Health,

found that the liver membranes of obese mice had fewer insulin receptors than those of lean mice, and that they took up only a little more than of a third of the insulin than did the membranes of lean mice. This suggested another link between obesity and diabetes.

At Stanford University, Olevsky and Reaven showed that blood cells taken from maturity-onset diabetics had approximately half as many receptors as cells taken from healthy individuals, and that they took up only about half the insulin.

Other findings suggested that there is an inverse link between the level of circulating insulin and the number of insulin receptors in liver, muscle, fat, and blood cells—the higher the level of circulating insulin, the fewer the receptors.

Just what causes the reduction in the number of receptors is still to be determined. Some research has indicated that obesity is linked to a reduction in receptors, while weight loss results in a receptor increase. There may be genetic factors. Certainly a number of questions remain to be answered, and the answers are being sought by a growing number of scientists. Hopefully, the problem of insulin resistance and its correction may be on its way to solution.

Another line of research has provided what may prove to be an important diagnostic test for beta cell tumors (insulinomas) and abnormal insulin elevations which cannot be measured by standard methods because of interference by circulating insulin antibodies. This finding is a tangential development from the discovery in 1967 of proinsulin by D. F. Steiner and P. E. Oyer. Proinsulin, a precursor of insulin, is a large molecule consisting of the insulin A and B chains connected by a group of amino acids known as a peptide. Proinsulin itself is inactive, and it is only when the peptide link is broken and chains A and B separated that the insulin becomes active. Because of its function as a link, the peptide is known as connecting- or C-peptide. By measuring the levels of C-peptide which are released into the circulation along with active insulin, Drs. D. L. Horwitz, H. Kuzuya, and A. H. Rubenstein of the University of Chicago found that they had a means of making an accurate measurement of actual circulating levels of insulin, regardless of the possible presence of insulin-binding antibodies.

A C-peptide kit has now been developed for physicians, and it seems likely that it will be used in demonstrating the remission or recovery phase of diabetes as well as in evaluating so-called brittle diabetics and the determination of hypoglycemic states.

In a further development, Rubenstein has reported the detection of C-peptide in some insulin-dependent diabetics, suggesting that these patients retain an insulin-producing capability.

Hemoglobin Provides Accurate Test

Blood sugar levels usually vary from moment to moment, depending upon food intake, physical activity, stress, and other factors. For this reason, the standard blood sugar tests provide a very narrow picture of the metabolic situation—they can indicate only the glucose level at the time the blood is drawn. They do not offer an extended view of the patient's ability to handle glucose—his or her general situation over a period of time—information that would permit reasonably accurate monitoring of the effectiveness of treatment as well as the relationship between the underlying diabetes and its complications.

This testing gap was apparently closed in 1976 when

Drs. C. Peterson, A. Cerami, M. Lehrman, and Q. Saudek of New York reported the development of a test which can show the state of diabetic control over a period of weeks or even months. They found that a particular type of hemoglobin (Hb A_{Ic}), the oxygen-carrying component of blood, increases as blood sugar levels rise, and decreases as blood sugar falls. However, the hemoglobin rises and falls at a slower rate, tending to reflect the average sugar levels over a period of time. Consequently, a single hemoglobin measurement will be able to indicate the degree of diabetes control far more accurately than the present methods. In turn, this improved accuracy should make correlations between control and the development of complications more meaningful than they are at present.

Beyond these factors, which can be put to prompt use in treating diabetics, the work with hemoglobin carries interesting implications that should spur further research: If blood sugar elevations are linked to a rise in oxygen-carrying hemoglobin, it would seem that the oxygen-carrying capacity of the hemoglobin itself may be reduced, requiring more hemoglobin to transport the required amount of oxygen.

New Approach to Complications Therapy

Continuing research by Dr. K. H. Gabbay of Harvard Medical School has opened a door to a possible means of treating and perhaps even preventing diabetic cataracts and neuropathies. Working under a grant from the Juvenile Diabetes Federation, he has found a way of blocking the formation of a sugar alcohol called sorbitol which, by accumulating in vulnerable cells, is involved in the development of cataracts and neuropathy.

Sorbitol is formed by the action of an enzyme, aldose

reductase, on glucose. In diabetics, abnormal amounts of glucose are thus converted into sorbitol, which then moves into the cells. What Gabbay and his associates have found and tested in experimental animals is that the conversion of glucose to sorbitol can be stopped by inhibiting the action of the enzyme that performs the conversion. This is done by administering a new drug, Alrestatin, which blocks the aldose reductase enzyme.

Following successful tests with animals, Gabbay began working with human volunteers in 1976, and early reports indicate success in treating some neuropathies. He is also conducting studies on the effect of Alrestatin on carbohydrate tolerance in normal individuals, juvenile diabetics, asymptomatic diabetics, and newly diagnosed diabetics in the remission phase. A particular point of interest is whether Alrestatin can accelerate the start of remission which is often seen in juvenile diabetics, and, certainly no less important, whether it can prolong the remission.

The answers, which will require careful and extended testing, can have a profound effect on the treatment of diabetes.

Increasing the Insulin Supply

The development of new approaches to the treatment of diabetes, particularly insulin-dependent diabetes, has been a problem of growing concern. Diabetes, as we have seen, touches an increasing number of people each year. In the United States alone some 10 million people were affected by diabetes in 1973. The prevalence of the disease increased by 50 percent between 1965 and 1973, and if this increase in the number of diabetics is matched, as expected, by an increased demand for insulin, the rising cost of animal insulin is certain to become a serious problem.

The most immediately obvious solution is the synthesis of insulin, thus breaking free of the dependence upon the limited population of livestock. Despite some extremely complex problems, considerable progress has been made in this area, and a group of German scientists appear to have brought us to the point where commercial synthesis of insulin is feasible.

A number of monumentally difficult tasks had to be accomplished along the way. First, F. Sanger of Cambridge, England, had to unravel the incredibly complicated insulin molecule and reveal its structure. This led to the partial, and then final, synthesis of the insulin A and B chains and their linkage by the Toronto group of G. H. Dixon, Y. C. Du and his colleagues in Shanghai and Peking, H. Zahnd in Aachen, and the Pittsburgh team of P. G. Katsoyannis.

Unfortunately, although the way to synthesis was open, only small amounts could be produced, and at very great expense. Then, in 1975, a further advance in synthesis was announced by the German pharmaceutical company Hoechst, which reported that one of its scientists, R. Obermeier, in collaboration with Zahnd, had apparently solved most of the problems and that commercial production of synthetic insulin would soon be possible.

Pancreatic Transplants

One major problem with drug therapy of diabetes, regardless of whether insulin or other agents are used, is that the treatment does not provide the minute-by-minute balance required by the body's constantly changing metabolic needs. Normally, the pancreas and liver answer the demands of the body as they occur, releasing just enough glucose, glucagon, and somatostatin to maintain the body at a steady state. Unfortunately, such fine regulation is impossible with injected insulin or other antidiabetes drugs. It is for this reason that perfect control of diabetes is not yet possible. Regardless of how careful and expert the treatment, there will be moments when the patient's blood sugar will be either a little too high or a little too low, depending upon the timing and dosage of the drug taken, the timing and content of the last meal, physical activity, stress, and so on.

Theoretically, of course, the best solution for an insulin-dependent patient would be a new pancreas. This was attempted late in 1966 by Dr. R. C. Lillehei and his colleagues at the University of Minnesota. After that first recorded pancreatic transplant, 46 others were performed in the following 10 years. Of those patients, only one was alive at the end of 1975. The difficulties were very great and the rejection rate very high.

Islet Cell Transplants

Meanwhile, researchers were trying other solutions. Some scientists had demonstrated that it was not necessary to transplant the entire pancreas, which, since it also secreted digestive enzymes that had to be diverted, created additional surgical problems. Instead, they showed that it was enough to transplant the islets of Langerhans, which could actually be injected.

Some of the most important work in this area was performed by Dr. P. E. Lacy and his group at Washington University in St. Louis, Dr. C. F. Barker at the University of Pennsylvania, Dr. J. Brown at U.C.L.A., and Dr. J. S. Najarian at the University of Minnesota.

The critical task, performed by Lacy and his team, was

to show that the islets could be isolated from the other pancreatic tissues. However, the recovery rate was low, with an average of slightly less than 450 islets being recovered from a rat pancreas that normally contains approximately 15,000 islets. Since anywhere from 500 to 2400 islets are generally used for each experimental injection, the problem becomes obvious.

Lacy found that the most effective site for the islet injection was the portal vein of the liver. The islet cells gather in the branches of the vein, acquire a blood supply, and begin releasing insulin directly into the liver, where insulin is believed to perform its primary role.

Rats made diabetic by the removal or destruction of the pancreas were able to maintain normal blood sugar levels for a year or more following a single islet cell injection. The rejection rate of islet cells seems lower than that for the whole pancreas, particularly if they are injected into the portal vein. If the islet cells are taken from fetuses, they are tolerated even longer.

While virtually all the work has been done with animals, both Lacy and Najarian have isolated human islets. The human pancreas contains about a million or more islets, and it is estimated that anywhere from 50,000 to 100,000 will be required for a graft. Najarian injects the islets directly into the peritoneum, a procedure which requires a greater number of islets than the portal site but does not involve a surgical incision to expose the portal vein. Grafts have been made in some diabetic patients, and the initial results seem very promising. However, more time and much more experience are needed before the value of this procedure can be judged.

The Artificial Pancreas

Another approach to the problem is the creation of an artificial pancreas. This is not a new idea. In 1962, A. H.

Kadish of Los Angeles combined an auto-analyzer, to measure glucose levels, with equipment that would inject either glucose or insulin as needed. While this combination of devices was too cumbersome to be practical, it did show that an approach combining continuous monitoring and glucose/insulin infusion as required was feasible as well as useful.

Improvements on the Kadish artificial pancreas have been made in a number of centers. In Toronto, Drs. B. S. Liebel and A. M. Albisser used autoanalyzer and glucose/insulin injection devices in combination with computers which control blood sugar levels according to strict mathematical formulas. They, along with Dr. E. F. Pfeiffer, in West Germany, have shown that this artificial pancreas, developed by the Ames Company, can do better than standard insulin injections in maintaining normal blood sugar levels. However, the device is still quite large and consequently can be used only in a hospital setting. There it has shown its worth in overcoming diabetic coma swiftly and safely, and in controlling diabetes in surgical patients.

The bulk of the artificial pancreas is due in great part to the autoanalyzer, which serves as the sensor that measures blood sugar levels. In order to reduce the size of the overall device, scientists and engineers are currently working on the miniaturization of sensors.

A sensor about the size of a quarter has been developed by Dr. J. S. Soeldner and his group at Boston's Joslin Clinic, acting in cooperation with a team from the Whittaker Corporation.

Thus far, the smallest sensor, about the size of a five-cent piece, has been developed by Dr. S. E. Bessman and his associates at the University of Southern California.

All three of these sensors use somewhat differing methods to provide continuous measurement of blood sugar levels. All have been tested in animals and have apparently performed well. However, a miniaturized sensor, while a great step forward, is not yet an artificial pancreas. A miniaturized insulin/glucose infusion device must be combined with the sensor to give it pancreatic-type function—and the combined instrument should be small enough for the diabetic to carry comfortably.

Such an artificial pancreas may not be too far off. Bessman, in conjunction with Dr. L. J. Thomas, has developed a miniaturized pump capable of delivering insulin. This has been combined with the sensor and a tiny computer that translates sensor information into instructions for the pump, along with a battery, into a package about 50 cc in size. This is small enough to be implanted.

Of course, many serious problems remain with the artificial pancreas: the continuing efficiency of the delicate sensor apparatus, the precise operation of the pump, the extent of battery life. Somewhat similar problems with the cardiac pacemaker were met and solved. Presumably, solutions to the problems of the artificial pancreas will also be found.

But will the artificial pancreas, when it is perfected, be able to perform the function of the normal pancreas in maintaining and adjusting carbohydrate metabolism according to the body's needs? And, if it indeed accomplishes this, will the complications of diabetes be prevented?

While this key question remains to be answered, a possible clue has been provided by Najarian, at least as far as islet transplants are concerned. He demonstrated that following islet cell transplants into rats with diseased kidneys, the kidney disease was relieved.

Since the artificial pancreas should perform a function similar to that of the grafted islets, it is not inconceivable that the device might well prevent the often serious complications associated with diabetes.

Altogether, the research prospects are very hopeful.

For thousands of years our knowledge of diabetes was frozen by ignorance and the prejudice it engendered. Today there is vigorous activity on a world scale. All aspects of diabetes are involved in the research, from basic causes to new forms of therapy and possible prevention.

We may not yet have mastered diabetes, but we have learned to control it. We can detect it, treat it, curb its symptoms, reduce its complications, and cope with most of its problems. What is more, these things can be done with a minimum of intrusion into the ordinary routines of daily living.

Consequently, whatever promises are still to be fulfilled, today's diabetic can live a fuller, longer, and more nearly normal life than was ever before imagined possible.

Index